THAT'S WHAT JUNKIES DO

Thomas M. Figlioli

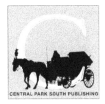

CENTRAL PARK SOUTH PUBLISHING

Publisher: Central Park south Publishing
Website: www.centralparksouthpublishing.com

Publisher's Note: True Story, Non-Fiction.

Book Layout: Victor Marcos

THAT'S WHAT JUNKIES DO by Thomas M. Figlioli – 1st ed. © 2021
ISBN: 978-1-7370777-0-1

CONTENTS

Acknowledgments

Thank you to everyone that never gave up on me. Thank you mom and Stephanie for being there for me no matter how bad things got. I would not be the man I am today without your unconditional love and support. Thank you Little Chris, Sean, Anna, Greggy and the rest of the KIF crew, we will always have that basement. Thank you John for answering the phone on that cold January day. Thank you to the staff at Mirmont Treatment Center. You guys nursed me back to health when I was physically, mentally and spiritually at my worst. The staff and the community gave me the jumpstart I needed to be where I am today. Thank you to "my friend" Dennis. This book started out with me writing a few stories and ideas in my I Phone notepad. Your reaction after reading them and subsequent encouragement gave me the confidence to turn it into something more. Thank you to everyone I have come across in the Staten Island recovery community, especially my Cleveland Ave people. You made me feel at home from day one and I am grateful to you all. Thank you Mario for loving me like a son and challenging me to be better. Thank you Rose, Mario, Sal and Pa for accepting me into your family. Thank you Jen and Nicky for being the brother and sister I never had and two of my biggest supporters. Thank you Nicky and Dom for being the craziest little people I ever met. Being your uncle, while exhausting at times, is one of the greatest blessings in my life. Last but most certainly not least I want to thank my beautiful wife Diana. You are my best friend, my biggest cheerleader and there is nobody I would rather do life with. All your support and encouragement along the way made it possible for me to write this book. I am eternally grateful that God put you in my life and I will love you forever.

THAT'S WHAT JUNKIES DO

It was early 2003 and the night like any other over the last three years. We were hanging out in G's basement drinking beers and smoking weed. By now, alcohol and drugs had caused a lot of problems in my life. I had been a daily drinker since I was seventeen, a cocaine addict since twenty - three and an opiate addict for the last year. I wore out my welcome in Westchester and had to move back to Brooklyn with my family. I lost two jobs, one being a promising career in the financial industry. At twenty-seven years old I had already been locked up in a psych ward and cycled in and out of various outpatient programs as a direct result of drinking and using drugs.

On this night, a one-hundred-dollar bill went missing from G's basement. By now, it was becoming clear to my family and friends, that if money or pills were missing it was probably me. My friends never really confronted me. I guess they didn't want to believe the guy they all grew up with would steal from them like he didn't know them at all. That night however, G confronted me about the hundred dollars. Me, being the person that I was at the time, denied any knowledge of it. I argued that it wasn't me, that I would never do something like that. My other friends sat in silence. G was never afraid to speak his mind and was always the first one to speak up about my obvious issues.

"Tommy, where's my fucking hundred dollars? It was right there this morning, and now it's gone." He screamed.

"G, come on man. I would never steal from you. We know each other since we've been kids. I would never do that to you. You should know that. You should know me." I replied.

"I do know you Tommy. You steal from your mother, you steal from your aunt, those people raised you." He said with increasing disgust in his voice.

I was silent, I didn't know how to react. All I could do is what I've been doing since I was a kid and that was lie.

"G, I swear to God Man, I swear on my father's ashes, it wasn't me." I said with a hint of desperation in my voice.

"It was you Tommy. It was you because you steal from your family, you steal from your friends. It's because you're a junkie Tommy and that's what Junkies do."

I've never been shot or stabbed, but I can't imagine it feeling much worse than that. One of my best friends just said what had been the elephant in the room for the past few years. I was angry and I felt betrayed. How could he say those things about me? I wanted to scream at him. I wanted to hit him. At the same time I wanted to crawl under the couch and die because deep down I knew he was right. There were five people in the room that night. They all felt the same way, but he said it and now the cat was out of the bag. I did take that hundred dollars and I bought cocaine with it earlier that day. I also stole five 80 milligram Oxycontin from my aunt an hour after that. After a few moments of silence, I was asked to leave. I would get up and leave the uncomfortably silent basement that I hung out in every night for the last three years. I tearfully walked across the street to my house. That would be the last time I was welcome in my friend's home. I took that four hundred milligrams of Oxycontin. I snorted the hundred dollars worth of cocaine and I drank eighteen Coronas by myself that night.

The party was long over by that point and I was the junkie he said I was. There wasn't enough alcohol or drugs to make me forget what my life had become. I would do anything and hurt anyone for my next fix. It didn't matter who you were. More often than not, it was those closest to me that bore the brunt of my insanity. Over the next two years I would cross every line I said I wouldn't. I would lose everything and everyone I ever cared about because chasing a high and numbing the pain became the most important thing in my life. I didn't want to do it anymore, and thoughts of taking my own life grew stronger with each passing day.

When people think of a drug addict or an alcoholic, they think of the mugshots. They think of the people they see living on the streets, or on the news getting locked up for a crime they committed in furtherance of their addiction. They think of the body lying in the morgue, just another junkie that threw away their life chasing death for a feeling. Jails, death and institutions are the three end games for the addict that doesn't change their ways, but that's not how it starts. My story is not much different than anyone else who struggles with addiction. The substances and circumstances may be different. The times and places may be different. The one thing they all have in common is that they are all stories of progression. I started out as an innocent kid. I had dreams and aspirations until alcohol and drugs took it all away. As I lay in my bed that night, I couldn't help but look back at my life. Where did it all go wrong? Why did I end up the way I did? I wish I could say that night was the end of my struggle, but it wasn't. Things would get worse before they ever got better. There would be more heartache and pain. I would hurt myself and everyone close to me before I finally took that first step to turning it all around. This is my story.

CHAPTER 1

The Beginning

I grew up in Brooklyn, Ny in the 80's and early 90's. I lived in a two-family home in a small private court on the border of Borough Park and Dyker Heights, a neighborhood full of Italian and Irish families. You could always find someone outside to play ball, cause mischief or simply shoot the shit with. I loved my early childhood and have nothing but fond memories of it. My father was full blooded Italian, and my mother was Irish. When I was six years old my mother's sister and two older cousins moved in to our second floor apartment and I was thrilled. I loved my aunt like a mother and my cousins became the brother and sister I never had. My father wasn't too happy because he couldn't charge the rent he wanted to, but he sucked it up and we lived as one big happy family, or so I thought.

My mother went back to work when I was around ten years old for Long Island College Hospital. She was a hard worker, who took pride in everything she did. My father was a street guy. He owned several businesses during my childhood, one being a very successful car service in Sheepshead Bay. My father had a golden tongue, or the gift of gab, as my mother puts it, and he always had "friends" helping him out along the way. He could take any business and turn it to gold. He was also into various illegal activities such as loan sharking and bookmaking. The problem with my dad, was that he was a degenerate gambler and as a result often got in over his head with the people he associated with. I knew what a point spread was by the time I was five years old from sitting with him on Sunday mornings during football season. This caused a lot of tension between my parents and they would fight a lot, not talking to each other for days, sometimes weeks at a time. I didn't know then, but I would later find out the extent of his gambling and other misdeeds and it would cause a big rift in our relationship. Even with the constant tension between my parents I had a great childhood. Whatever problems they had with each other were never taken out on me. I was an only child and as far back as I can remember I was very spoiled. We would go on two vacations every year. It was Montauk every summer with Aunt Pat and Uncle Jim and the Nevele in upstate New York every winter with Aunt Grace, Uncle Tony and other friends of the family. My father would take me to sporting events and movies all the time and my mother thought of me as a little king and treated me as such. Whatever I wanted, whenever I wanted it, all I had to do was ask. My name is Tommy. Everyone calls me Tommy Figs or just plain old Figs, a short version of my last name. That's how it's been since that first time I stepped out of my house. Some older kid asked me my name and when I told him, I immediately became Figs, Figgy, Fig Newton and all the other variations of the name. Now, at forty-five years old, it still follows me. I have come to accept and even love it.

Growing up, I was a small skinny kid, shy around new people and passive for the most part. I had a great group of friends who all lived within ten houses of each other. Then there were the older kids. At the time it seemed like they were grown men, but they were only four or five years older than my group. These kids were tough. They liked to do the same things we did but they also liked to fight. They were loud, aggressive and had no problem throwing down whenever it was necessary. One summer day we were all outside playing ball and one of the older kids called me over to their group. I was about seven or eight years old at the time. They handed me a plastic bat, the long skinny yellow ones you could buy in any store back then. It was packed full of wet newspaper and wrapped in black electric tape, having the weight and feel of a regular aluminum baseball bat. Our street was divided into two courts, separated by a seven-foot-tall, sidewalk to sidewalk length black iron fence with a small opening to walk through if you contorted your body to measure three feet tall. The other court might as well have been another country and kids from that side weren't one of us. One of them pointed towards the other court.

"You see that kid over there. I want you to go hit him in the head with this bat." He said, as the rest of them egged me on.

In that moment, a million thoughts went through my head. I knew it was wrong, but this was a test to see how tough I was. I mean this kid was huge. At eight years old Tommy T was six feet tall and weighed about two hundred pounds. The fear and insecurity of the older kids not accepting me took over. I walked to the other court, went straight up to Tommy T, looked up and took my best swing right off the side of his head. As big as he was, I think deep down inside he felt smaller than me. He wasn't tough and he didn't deserve what I did to him, but I did it anyway. Tommy started crying and ran in his house. I ran back to the older kids and they were all laughing and commenting how nuts I was. I felt a sense of acceptance and pride in that moment, but that quickly changed to guilt and shame for what I did to him.

I went home and about an hour later my doorbell rang and my mother answered. It was Tommy and his dad. His dad wasn't happy at all and let my mother know what a rotten thing I did to his son. All my mother did was look at me and say, *"wait until your father gets home."* I dreaded those words. My father was an intimidating man. He never hit me because he didn't have to. One look was all it took to put the fear of God in me. The next few hours in my room felt like an eternity. Around seven o'clock I heard the gate open and I looked outside. I saw his big white Cadillac parked in front of the house like every other night, but this night was different. In his thick Brooklyn accent, he called up to me.

> *"Tommy"* He yelled.
> *"Yea dad"* I answered sheepishly.
> *"Get down here."*

I went down the stairs fully expecting a good crack.

> *"Come on, we're going for a ride."* He said as he walked toward the back door.

As I was walking behind him through the kitchen into the garage, I looked back at my mother to save me. She just looked at me and made a facial expression like, hey you brought this on yourself, it's out of my hands. We got in the car and there were no words spoken. Oldies music was playing in the car and he just stared straight ahead. His silence and the anticipation of what was to come next was enough to make me want to throw up. We drove for about fifteen minutes, but to me it seemed like four hours. We parked and he shut the car off. He turned to me and with his eyes staring over his glasses that were hanging slightly off his nose he started questioning me.

> *"What happened Tom?"* He said with subtle force in his voice.
> *"I hit the kid in the head with a wiffle bat dad."* I replied.
> *"Why did you do that?"* He asked.

I couldn't tell him the truth here. I had to think fast, and I did.

> *"He made fun of mommy and pushed me."* I said with a sense of urgency in my voice.

"Oh yea" He replied, seeming surprised.

"Yea dad"

"Who's this kid?" He curiously asked.

"Big Tommy T dad, from the other Court." I replied.

"You mean that kid that's bigger than me?" He said, sounding even more surprised.

"Yea dad."

"Ok come on, let's go. " He said with a gasp as he shifted to open the car door.

We got out of the car and walked into a small diner. We walked to the back and there were four guys sitting there. I recognized them as my father's friends. What happened next is something I wasn't expecting and something I never forgot. Instead of yelling at me, my father beaming with pride, proceeded to tell his friends what I did. They all sat there just like the older kids and laughed and said how nuts I was. My father looked at me and said,

"What kind of shake do you want ya little dick?" He asked.

"Vanilla dad" I replied.

"Vanilla, huh, just like your mother. " He said jokingly.

"Listen, if your mother ask's, I yelled at you and you'll never do it again, understand. "

"Yea dad, I understand."

I sat there for an hour with my dad and his friends all gushing over the fact that I stood up for my mother to a kid twice my size. There were no repercussions and no punishments. It was the exact opposite. That shame and guilt turned back into pride and a feeling of acceptance. My father was proud of me. If there was anybody I wanted approval from, more than the older kids on the block, it was my father.

That night, at a very young age, I came to three conclusions. The first one is that my father was a very different kind of man and father than my friend's dads. Two was that, when in doubt, lie your ass off. The third conclusion and probably the one that would lead to most of my struggles later in life was that being accepted means you sometimes do things, even if they're wrong, even if you don't want to. To be accepted by the people I wanted to be accepted by, I would sometimes have to be a different person than I really was. This surely was not a normal way to think but it's something that followed me through childhood and most of my adult life.

CHAPTER 2

Say It Ain't So

It was a cool September morning in 1989 and it was my first day of High School. I graduated from Regina Pacis elementary school that summer and was starting my freshman year at Xaverian High School in Bay Ridge, Brooklyn. Xaverian was an all-boys Catholic School that was known for its high academic and athletic standards as well as its discipline. My friend Brian and Steven from grade school were going there also so we decided to take the bus together. We didn't want to get dropped off by our parents on the first day. I mean we were 13, we were practically adults. As soon as we realized that we could sleep an extra half hour by getting a ride from our parents that whole "we were adults" attitude went right out the window. I was excited for the new experience but scared at the same time fear and uncertainty coursed through my veins, giving me an uneasy feeling. The questions ran through my head.

> *Would I make any friends?*
> *Would the classes be too hard?*
> *How are the older kids going to treat me?*

There it was again, the insecurity and fear of not being accepted. It was something I had early on in life, and it continued with every new endeavor.

My first day was relatively uneventful. I met a few new guys in my home room and had some small talk, but it was just a basic introduction to the school and what was to be expected of us. The one thing I did was sign up to try out for the Baseball team. It's something me and my father had been preparing for since we had our first catch together. I was a slick fielding lefty first baseman coming off my best year in Little League where my bat was finally starting to catch up with my glove. The first round of tryouts were being held on the following Monday, and I was ready.

Monday came, and I woke up ready to go. The school day couldn't end fast enough. A week in and I was already getting used to the daily routine of high school and had made a couple of new friends. When the bell rang, I sped to my locker grabbed my bag and changed into my baseball gear. The field we would be trying out on was about thirty blocks from school, so my father was outside to pick me up and take me. I think he was more excited than I was. We got to the field and there were about fifty or sixty kids warming up, doing stretches and throwing the ball around. My father wished me luck and down the hill I went, eventually taking my spot at first base. Ground ball after ground ball, throw after throw, high, low, soft or hard, I ate up everything. I was never worried about my fielding. I knew nobody could touch me on that end. Next came batting practice. We were all given ten pitches to show our stuff and I made solid contact with everything. I wasn't a power hitter, but I hit line drives all over the field. I felt like I did enough to make the first cut and so did my father, who along with being supportive, was also my harshest critic. The list was going to be posted on Tuesday afternoon and the daylong wait took forever. The wait was worth it as I made the first cut. The competition for first base was down to me and two other guys. The second round of tryouts would be on Thursday and I was cautiously optimistic that if I repeated my first performance it would be enough to make the team.

Thursday came and it was the same routine. I was struggling to sit still in class all day long with my nerves getting the best of me.

The bell rang and I was off. Dad drove me to the field again and I went down the hill to warm up with the rest of the kids that made it to the second round. There was more pressure today because it was the final cut. This day the drills was a lot more thorough, we did more throwing and running, neither one was a strong suit of mine. I did my thing during infield drills and when my turn at bat came, I hit the ball solidly once again. The two kids I was up against were monsters compared to me. They both stood six feet tall and hit with power. In the field neither could touch me, but first base is a power position and they both crushed me in that department. My hope was that they would take one of them as the starter and take me as a backup and late game defensive specialist. My father agreed that I did enough to make the team and even had a coach from another school in the area watching with him confirm both of our opinions. I would have to wait until Monday to find out if I made the team and the next three days would be the longest of my young life.

Monday came and the list would be up by the end of the day. I couldn't eat all day because the butterflies were having a party in my stomach. The final bell rang, and thirty young boys all rushed to the school bulletin board at once. There was laughing and high fiving. There were also a few looks of disappointment. The suspense was killing me as I made my way through the crowd to look at the board. In those few moments there were thoughts rushing through my young mind. I thought of how proud my father was going to be when I told him I made it, I thought of my mother crying tears of joy when I burst through the front door telling her I was on the team. I saw myself in the school's pinstripe uniform with the number seventeen that I wore for my favorite baseball player Keith Hernandez proudly displayed on my back. Finally, I imagined getting the game winning hit in my first game as a Clipper, my teammates mobbing me as I pumped my fist rounding first base, as my family and friends cheered from the bleachers. Those thoughts quickly disappeared when I made it to the front of the crowd. My name wasn't there. The two other kids made the team, and I did not. I stared at that board for what seemed to be twenty minutes, it had to be a mistake. A note on the bottom of the sheet of paper with all the names on it read;

"Congratulations to all the New members of the 1989-90 Freshman Baseball Team and thank you to all those who tried out. We welcome all of you to come back and try again next season. Have a great school year. GO CLIPPERS!!!"

It wasn't a mistake. My best wasn't good enough and I didn't make the team. My eyes instantly welled up and my throat started to close. I couldn't cry in front of everybody because I would be labeled a cry baby and a loser. I quickly ran to the bathroom and into the first open stall slamming the door behind me. I cried as quietly as I could. All the thoughts of mom and dad being proud turned to thoughts of how disappointed they would both be. I was supposed to play High School baseball and now that dream was dead. During the week of tryouts I was so determined and focused on the task at hand that there was no room for insecurity and fear. Even when I saw those guys crushing balls off the hill, I knew I put forth my best effort and I was confident that was enough. When that was all over the insecurity came back immediately. I went home that night and broke the news to my parents. They could tell just by looking at me that I hadn't made it. My mother was supportive and nurturing as usual encouraging me that the hurt wouldn't last forever and there'd be other teams and other tryouts.

"Just practice hard and build yourself up and next year you'll be on that team." She said.

I appreciated the words, but in that moment, I couldn't really buy in to what she was telling me. The disappointment was too fresh. My father tried to be supportive in his own way, which consisted of yelling a lot. He blamed the coach who he had a personal beef with. He blamed the vice principal's son who undeservingly made the team because of his last name. He blamed everybody and everything else he could because he couldn't accept the fact that I didn't make it because the other guys were better. I think he meant well, but all that really did was encourage me to fall into the habit of blaming others when things didn't go my way. Looking back, I wish he just patted me on the back and said good try son, we'll get them next year, but that wasn't his way, and the pressure he would put on me over the next few years to live up to unrealistic expectations was a big factor in our eventual strained relationship.

Things settled down in the following weeks and months. The disappointment from not making the baseball team slowly faded away and I made friends with a bunch of new guys. I started playing intramural roller hockey after school and most of those guys played for the schools Ice Hockey team. My father was putting constant pressure on me to get back to baseball and it was getting tiring. I loved playing, and it was a lot of fun, but he was turning it into something I dreaded. I was starting to get better at hockey and my new friends were encouraging me to try out for the team the following year. I could play on roller skates, but I had only been on ice skates once and it wasn't a pretty sight. I decided I was going to give it a shot, so my mother bought me all new hockey equipment and I dedicated myself one hundred percent to learning how to translate my game from concrete to ice. Months of skating lessons and a summer long hockey camp paid off and in September of my sophomore year I became a member of the JV Ice Hockey team. It was the proudest moment of my life to that point. I set my mind on something I wanted and busted my ass to get it. I gave up baseball and became a fulltime hockey player splitting time between my ice hockey team and two local roller hockey teams. My decision to give up baseball was partly due to my father's insane pressure, but it was also because I just liked playing hockey more. He wasn't happy about it, but he learned to accept it and eventually support it. All things being equal, my sophomore year and first season as a hockey player was one of the best times of my life.

CHAPTER 3

Until We Meet Again

Junior year was at Xaverian was a good year. I did well academically and I moved up to the varsity hockey team. While my season wasn't as good as the year before, my play was steadily improving and I looked forward to ending my hockey career at Xaverian on a good note the following year. The summer between junior and senior year however, was one that would change my life forever. My father's gambling, and infidelity was out of control and now I was old enough to know what was going on. I hated being around him and our relationship became almost non-existent. I spent most of my time down at my friend's house and whenever I was home, I was upstairs in my cousin's room playing video games. One afternoon while was sleeping on his recliner, I tried to sneak by him so I could get up to my aunt's house without having to talk to him. He must have heard me going up the stairs because he called up to me.

"Hey, where are you going?" My father asked.
"Upstairs Dad" I replied.
"What else is new, you're going to play those goddamn games again." He said with disgust in his voice.

I didn't even answer him because I felt that he wasn't worth my time and energy.

"You know what, you really suck as a son." He said in the most hurtful way possible.

Those words cut through me like a knife. How could the man I idolized as a young boy say that to me? I did everything I could to gain his approval, to make him proud, and it all meant nothing to him. I never cursed at either one of my parents, but in that moment while holding back tears I couldn't keep it in.

"Go fuck yourself dad, you miserable bastard." I yelled back at him.

I went upstairs and cried. I felt bad for saying that to him, but I was hurt. It had been building for a long time and I exploded. I wish I handled it differently but just like his words to me, I couldn't take it back. The truth is, he deserved it. I had a long talk with my mother that night and she finally broke down and told me a great deal of what had been going on for the last sixteen years. The more she told me the angrier I became. How could he do these things to my mother, to our family. There were so many things going through my head. All the vacations, the parties, the family gatherings were all a big show. The perfect family role they played was a cover for what was really going on. In that moment I felt like my whole life was a lie. What I said next surprised both of us.

"Throw him out mom, just throw him out." I said, holding back tears.

She looked at me with a sense of calm and relief, like she had been waiting for me to give her the ok to do what she has wanted to do for a long time. My mother had been holding it together for years just for the sake of me having a stable family. It was time for her to do the right thing for herself. We both cried. She hugged me for at least ten minutes, kissed me on the cheek and said;

"Don't worry honey, everything will be ok."

My mother would spend much of the next decade busting her ass to keep that promise. The next day I was outside on the court throwing the football around with a few friends. My father came outside and called me over.

"Tommy, come here." He yelled.
"What's up dad?"

I was still mad from his comments the day before, and the things my mother told me made me lose a lot of respect for him. I really didn't want to hear some bullshit apology or explanation that afternoon, but I went over to him anyway. What I got from him was something completely different.

"Come inside a minute." He said with a sound of defeat in his voice.

I followed him into the basement not sure where this was heading.

"I'm leaving Tom. Me and your mother had a talk, and she doesn't want me here anymore so I'm going to leave. I'm going to Mickey's house in Rockaway. If you need me, here's the number."

He handed me a piece of paper with his girlfriend's phone number on it and hugged me. I felt just as crushed as the day before when he told me I sucked as a son. Despite what our relationship had become he was still my father. He was still the first man I looked up to, and in that moment, I didn't want him to leave. I hugged him tight and we cried together. I watched him walk out the door through our back yard and out of my life. I was just about to turn seventeen and my father wouldn't be a big part of my life from that day on. A few years later my mother being the woman she is, invited him to Christmas dinner when he had nowhere to go. That night, my father made his amends to me. He said that he was sorry for everything he put me and my mother through and told me never to do the things he had done. I spent some time with him over the next two years trying to mend our relationship, but it was never the same. The phone rang on a summer morning in July of 1997 and my roommate handed me the phone. My father was found dead in his room at an assisted living residence in Staten Island. His fast lifestyle and physical ailments finally caught up to him. The official cause of death was congestive heart failure, but it was the years of gambling, lying, stealing and cheating that truly caused his life to be cut so short. With nobody left to take care of him he died alone in a small room with nothing left in his life. He was sixty-one years old.

It wasn't until much later in life and my journey in recovery that I truly understood him. My father wasn't a bad man, he was a sick man. His gambling addiction and serial infidelity led him to live his life in a way that hurt himself and everybody around him. His over-the-top bravado and flashy lifestyle were a mask. Deep down inside, just like me, he was still an insecure little boy trying desperately to be accepted. I was able to identify and come to terms with that well into my thirties and finally forgive him.

Rest In Peace.
Vito Figlioli
4/15/36 – 7/15/97

CHAPTER 4

'84 Grand

The divorce of my parents changed the atmosphere at home. My father was no longer in the picture, but I still lived in a loving family household with my mother, aunt, and two cousins, who made sure I was well taken care of. Truth of the matter is that my mother had been supporting us for a long time now, so my father leaving really had no financial effect on us. With his negative presence no longer around it almost felt like the house was brighter. I was about to turn seventeen and start my senior year of high school. I was excited to start the new school year and leave that summer behind me. People were always asking me if I was ok and if I needed anything. One teacher who got some misinformation on my home situation even offered me a room in his house if things ever got too bad at home. I always replied with an "ok" and a smile, but I really wasn't ok. Learning that the man you looked up to for so long wasn't who you thought he was is a hard thing for a kid, especially at the age where you need a positive male influence the most.

One night right before school was about to start, a few of us were hanging out on my porch when I saw my friend Johnny. We had a falling out the previous summer over some stupid teenage love triangle involving him and my friend Mikey. Me and Johnny used to be tight, we played baseball together the year before we started high school with our fathers coaching the team. I would see him from time to time when he would visit his cousins who lived two doors down from me, but the friendship was never the same. He was walking with two girls from the neighborhood, but these weren't girls I was used to seeing on my block. These girls were from the Annex. The Annex was a board of ed building that had a big empty schoolyard that they used as a parking lot. We would play basketball and baseball there during the day with guys from all different parts of the neighborhood. At night, the Annex became a huge hangout. Some nights there would be a hundred people in there anywhere from fifteen to twenty-five years old hanging out drinking, smoking and God knows what else. I was always curious about the Annex, but my father always said if he ever caught me in there, he'd break my legs, plus, in all honesty the place scared the shit out of me.

So, Johnny is walking with his arms around these two annex girls. In one hand he has a cigarette and in the other he has a bottle of Budweiser. He looked up at me and my friends and gave a nod and a big smile like, *"look at what I got"*. Me and my friends all looked at each other in awe. There is no way we could ever talk to those girls. At that point of our lives the annex girls were way out of our league. We went on about our night talking about the upcoming school year and eventually wound up in my cousin's room playing video games. As the night went on, I couldn't stop thinking about Johnny with those girls. more importantly I couldn't get the image of the beer and cigarette he was holding out of my head. My cousin was thirteen years older than me and it wasn't a secret he smoked a lot of cigarettes and a lot of weed. That night while he was in the kitchen making a ham sandwich to satisfy his munchies, I stole one of his Marlboro Reds. I said I was tired and wanted to go to sleep early and went down to my house. I looked at that cigarette for an hour going back and forth in my head whether I should smoke it or not. It wasn't until that night, seeing Johnny with that cigarette, that I ever considered smoking. I went downstairs into the windowless bathroom we had in our basement. I stared in the mirror with this thing hanging from my lip, trying to look as cool as I could. I lit it up and took a small drag and nothing happened. I didn't cough, my chest didn't burn, absolutely nothing happened. I took a second drag, and there it was. It felt like I swallowed fire. The first drag was just the paper, the second one was chock full of tobacco. It was a good thing I was in the bathroom, because after I got done coughing my brains out, I got lightheaded and nauseous and threw up that night's dinner in the toilet. I threw the cigarette in the bowl, flushed it, washed my face and went to bed. My first experience with a cigarette was awful. I even ratted myself out to my mother and promised her I'd never take a puff of one again. That promise lasted about three weeks. A few weeks went by and school started. I still couldn't get the idea of Johnny and those two girls out of my head. I wanted to be able to talk to those girls. I wanted to hang out in the Annex, but I wasn't like those kids. They would laugh me out of that schoolyard the second I got there. One day in class I overheard two kids talking about hanging out that weekend. They were going to get some beer and go up to the Annex. Now these were regular kids. They weren't overly popular and they weren't athletes. They weren't even from the same neighborhood as me. Why could these kids go and not me? It became an obsession.

On a cool September morning in 1992 I was set to take the second round of my college entrance exams. Good grades and taking tests always came easy to me so I really wasn't nervous at all which was completely out of character for me. My friends and I had been preparing for the last few months, taking practice tests all summer and early fall. We made plans after the test to go to Caesars Bay Bazaar, a flea market type department store in Brooklyn that was a popular hangout for kids our age. We were all going to buy leather MC jackets so we could wear them to a party at my friend Patty's house later that night. His parents were on a cruise and when parents were away parties were thrown. This party was going to be different. My friend Mikey got his hands on a bottle of cheap Vodka and a bottle of Peach Schnapps. He suggested we do some shots before the party. None of us ever drank alcohol before and I knew it wasn't right, but I immediately thought of Johnny walking with the two girls and the beer. I thought of the two kids in class that Friday talking about getting beer and going to the Annex and my seventeen-year-old brain started to run away with itself. The only thing different about those kids in the class that Friday was the beer. The only thing different between me and Johnny was the beer. I'm in, were the next words that came out of my mouth. It's like an outside force took over my brain. I knew there would be consequences if I got caught, but in that moment I didn't care. It was just like that summer afternoon years earlier when I hit Tommy T with the bat. I knew then that I would sometimes have to do things to fit in even if I knew they were wrong. The kids in the Annex drank and if I wanted to be a part of that I had to drink as well.

That night we met in Mikey's house at seven o'clock. It was me, Mikey, Eric and Brian. We started off with a shot of vodka each. I hear a lot of people share at twelve step meetings that when alcohol first touched their lips, they got an instant feeling of ease and comfort. I can tell you that wasn't the case for this alcoholic. As soon as it hit my lips and went down my throat, I had to do everything in my power not to throw it back up. It was awful. We followed that up with a shot of Peach Schnapps. We took one more shot of Vodka and one more Schnapps. The Vodka went down a little easier this time, warming my chest as it made its way down my throat and into my stomach. It was time to go down to Patty's house for the party. I had a nice little buzz on. It was my first experience with alcohol, and I liked the feeling. When we got there, we started mingling and before I knew it, I was talking to a girl I had liked for a while but never had the nerve to approach. I didn't feel nervous. I didn't overthink it in my head. I saw her, walked over, and just said hello. I couldn't even tell you what else I said. I just remember her laughing and touching my arm and chest a lot. As I write this book I talk about fear, anxiety and insecurity quite often. I didn't know what those feelings were back then. I just knew I didn't feel quite right my whole childhood. I didn't take that first drink because of those feelings. I took it because I wanted to fit in with a certain group of people and felt I had to drink to do so. That sense of ease and comfort from the first shot I hear so much about didn't hit me until I started interacting with people out of my comfort zone. Without even realizing it, I felt comfortable. There was no fear. There was no insecurity. I wasn't thinking about my parents splitting up for the first time in months. For the first time in my life, I felt right.

The four of us left the party and we went back to Mikey's house to drink some more. We polished off the Schnapps between the four of us, then me Eric and Brian went out to Eric's car. We weren't old enough to drive yet, but Eric's dad bought him a 1984 silver Grand Prix for the day when he would eventually get his license. That car sat in front of their house which was directly across the street from mine for two years. We decided to hang out in the car and listen to music while we finished off the Vodka. We sat and listened to Guns N Roses and Bon Jovi for about an hour taking swigs from the bottle every few minutes and then decided to go back down to Patty's. Feeling no pain, we got out of Eric's car and that's when it happened. I was standing still but the street was moving. I tried walking straight, but it felt like someone was tilting the earth in front of me. I managed to make it down to Patty's house where his sister Kelly was outside smoking a cigarette with her friend. I saw three of each of them. I raised my hand to wave hello and that was apparently too much for my brain and body to handle. I collapsed face down onto the pavement like Mike Tyson just punched me in the jaw. The rest of the night is hazy at best. The two things I do remember are throwing up in the back seat of Eric's car and then Eric kicking me in the ribs for doing so. I can't say I blame him. The poor guys car smelled like Peach Schnapps and throw up for a year after that night.

I woke up the next day, completely disheveled, on the floor of my bedroom. I was fully clothed except for one sneaker that I never found. I went downstairs to feel out my mother and see if she suspected anything. There was nothing. She was in a very good mood, making me bacon and eggs. I got away with it. I felt like shit, my ribs were sore, and I had to buy new sneakers, but I got away with it. I got away with it, just like when I hit Tommy with the bat, and I couldn't wait to do it again. A week later I was up in the Annex, with Johnny, the two girls and a hundred other people smoking cigarettes and drinking beers. That's what alcohol did for me from the very start. It made me feel part of. Any insecurities I had were gone. The knot I had in my stomach every time I had to try something new or be around new people went away. It opened a whole new world for me. It gave me the ability to go into any situation without any fear of failure. The problem with that was that when I wasn't drinking, all that stuff was back, worse than before. The only thing that would make it better was to drink more. If I knew that Saturday night in October of '92 would be the start of a lifelong struggle, I may have never taken that first sip. My senior year of high school was spent hanging out in the Annex, going to house parties, school dances and bars that let underage kids in with no ID. I quit the hockey team a week into the season because hockey just got in the way of drinking and hanging out. I was still able to graduate near the top of my class and I was awarded The Deans Business Scholarship from Pace University. I decided to go to the Pleasantville Campus about an hour and fifteen minutes north of NYC. They were paying most of the way so why not get the full college experience and live away from home. I was about to start a new chapter of my life and I couldn't be more excited.

CHAPTER 5

We Were Merely Freshmen

It was the summer of 1993 and I was getting ready to start my freshman year of college in Pleasantville, Ny. By getting ready, I mean working at my cousin's brokerage firm during the day and drinking every night. It was going to be a while before I saw my friends again, so we were ending the summer with a blast. There were no real nerves about going away to school. The main reason for that was because I was drunk and stoned most of the time. The second was that I was going to be living with two guys from Xaverian that I had become close with senior year. Me and my friend Lou were set to be roommates when a mix up in the admissions department left both of us in single rooms. My friend Ciro was also going to Pace so to make up for their mistake they gave the three of us a quad with the promise they wouldn't fill the fourth spot.

The day came for us to move in. I was going to miss my friends from Brooklyn, but I was excited to live on my own for the first time. Me, mom and Aunt Eileen got there first. We were followed almost immediately by Lou and his dad. We were just hanging out talking when Ciro arrived. Ciro was seventeen but acted like he was forty-five. He was the most responsible kid I had ever met and everybody loved him. He was a lot of fun to be around when he wasn't yelling at you to pick up after yourself. Lou and I were Italian, but Ciro was ITALIAN!!! His family was right out of the movies. Me and Lou each had a representative or two from our families, but not Ciro. When the door opened, relative after relative walked through. Dad, mom, brother, sister, cousin, cousin, aunt, uncle and finally grandma. Grandma looked like she was going to a wake, dressed in all black with the veil over her face. She spoke to everybody in Italian whether you understood her or not. Each person had some sort of food with them and they all hugged and kissed you like they knew you for forty years. We always busted Ciro's chops about them, but the truth was, I thought it was awesome. There was thirty people in the room now, twenty of them Ciro's relatives, and we all ate and talked for the next two hours.

It was time for the families to leave and as we all said our goodbyes tears were shed, mostly by my mother. When the door finally shut as the last member of Ciro's entourage exited the room we all broke out our cigarettes and lit up. Here's to freedom, was the mood in the room. There was nobody to answer to, no curfews, no trying to hide anything. We were on our own and ready to take Pace Pleasantville by storm. We got settled in and did our mandatory orientation. Now it was time to find the parties and find them we did. We all got wrecked that first night. Ciro got the worst of it, throwing up all over himself during his drunk rendition of Sinatra's My Way. We made friends with a group of girls from the Bronx that first night and stayed friends with them and their families our entire time there. They were awesome girls, just like us, friends from high school trying to adapt to a new setting. The great thing about going away to college is that nobody knows you and you can reinvent yourself into whatever you want. All anybody knew was that we were three Italian kids from Brooklyn and they assumed every stereotype that goes along with that. We were more than happy to play along and it wasn't long before our room would become fondly known as Little Italy. That first night was a sign of things to come and Little Italy became the sight of many a late-night party. The thing about reinventing yourself is that you start to forget who you were in the first place. I compare it to developing a character in a movie or book. I would pick and choose traits from my favorite tv and movie characters and make them part of myself. I had been doing this since that first night in the Grand Prix. At first the alcohol made it easier to act a certain way without fear of rejection or ridicule. After a while the alcohol just became part of the character.

We quickly made friends in the dorm. Everybody wanted to hang out with the kids from Little Italy, especially Jeff. Jeff was a kid from Yonkers who didn't live on campus. Lou met him the first night and he passed out on the floor of our room. Jeff never left and he wound up becoming one of my best friends in the world. I still shoot Jeff a text every time I see a movie or hear a song that reminds me of our time at Pace. There were about twenty-five of us from the dorm. Rush season is when all the fraternities and sororities on campus recruit new members. There are different parties and events every night of the week. When rush season came around, we decided that we were all going to pledge the same fraternity. We picked Delta Upsilon because they were the coolest bunch of guys we met. They all seemed down to earth, they were non-secretive to a point, and most of them were upper classmen. If we all got in, the fraternity would be in our control within two years. We started pledging in early September and went all the way through to late November. Long story short we got in and we had a big celebration the night of initiation. It was a long, often grueling process, but we all stuck together and made it. There was a sense of accomplishment and pride among us and we proudly displayed our new letters around campus the following day.

By the way I'm already in late November and I haven't once mentioned school. I haven't mentioned studying for tests or writing papers. The reason for that is I didn't go to school. I spent twelve weeks pledging a fraternity. Twelve weeks drinking every night and sleeping all day. Twelve weeks entertaining my friends from Brooklyn who would come up for "two days" and stay three weeks. If I went to ten classes, it was a lot. There was another guy Jeff who was already a brother. He was a great guy who went on to become a Sergeant in the

NYPD, but he was a loud pain in the ass. He had the reputation of being the biggest and best drinker in the fraternity. I decided early on that I was going to take that title from him. I was there on scholarship with my mother working seven days a week to foot the rest of the bill. I had to maintain a 3.00 GPA and not get into any disciplinary jackpots, yet there I was putting all my energy into becoming a character from Animal House. My hard work paid off and I failed three classes, got a 1.62 GPA and almost got thrown off campus for destruction of property. The crowning jewel of my first semester was that I beat out Jeff for the coveted award of "*MOST LIKELY TO WIND UP IN AA*". I framed that certificate and displayed it proudly above my bed. I always used to think my life didn't start to unravel until much later in my story. My first semester at Pace was a sure sign that I was heading down the wrong path, but I was just a college kid doing what college kids do so nobody gave it a second thought.

I started the second semester on academic probation. The scholarship was gone either way because there was no mathematical way to get my GPA over a 3.0 for the year so I wrote a letter to the school saying how hard my parents' divorce had been on me. I told them that I really needed the financial support because my mother couldn't afford the full ride. They agreed that if I got a 3.0 for the second semester, they would give me a hardship grant in the same amount as the scholarship. Like most addicts and alcoholics, I did my best work when my back was against the wall. I mean I still drank every night, but I went to class most of the time. I did the papers, took the tests and got a 3.2 GPA. That got me the grant and got me off academic probation. Just like that I was back on track.

CHAPTER 6

MATTEAU!! MATTEAU!! MATTEAU!!

It was the spring of 1994 and the school year had just ended. Despite my best efforts to get kicked out of school my first semester I managed to redeem myself and I would be heading back to Little Italy at the end of the summer. I was going home for three months and I was excited to see my friends and catch up. My summer job at the brokerage firm was still there for me, so everything was in place for an enjoyable summer back in Brooklyn. The New York Rangers were on their Stanley Cup championship run and me and my friends gathered every night in my living room to watch the games. There are moments in your life that are permanently burned into your memory. The night of May 27, 1994 was one of those nights.

It was Game Seven of the Stanley Cup Eastern Conference Finals. The Rangers and Devils had battled back and forth for six epic games, most notably Ranger's Captain Mark Messier's Game Six guarantee and subsequent hat trick. The excitement in the day leading up to Game Seven was insane. Jeff was coming down from Yonkers to watch it with us, and we all met on my front porch ten minutes before game time. We were all superstitious, so we had to see the national anthem, sit in the same seats, and wear the same clothes as we wore when they won game six. It was a hard fought, intense, edge of your seat game. The kind so often seen in the Stanley Cup playoffs. Leading 1-0 heading into the final moments of the game we were all bursting at the seams, eager to celebrate the win that would send the Rangers to the finals for a chance to win their first cup in fifty-four years. The clock ticked to 7.7 seconds, and with their goalie pulled the Devils tied the game at one. It felt like the room was a big balloon and somebody just stuck a ten-foot pin in it. I vividly remember Jeff sitting on the top step leading to my basement repeatedly banging his head against wall. It was time for another overtime game. If you're a hockey fan, you know that sudden death overtime of a playoff game is like torture. Double overtime is even worse. Double OT in game seven is a gut wrenching feeling I can't even describe. We were physically and mentally exhausted as if we were playing the game ourselves. The second OT started and it was the typical back and forth. Then it happened. Four minutes and twenty-four seconds into the second overtime, it happened.

"Fetisov for the Devils plays it cross-ice, into the far corner. Matteau swoops in to intercept. Matteau behind the net, swings it in front. He scores! Matteau! Matteau! Matteau! Stephane Matteau! and the Rangers have one more hill to climb, baby, and it's Mount Vancouver! The Rangers are headed to the Finals!"

In what is still considered by many as the greatest call of a goal in NHL history, Ranger radio voice Howie Rose screamed with elation as Stefane Matteau scored the game winner. The Rangers were going to the finals. We went berserk, jumping up and down hugging each other to the point of my mother yelling at us not to come through the ceiling. That game and that moment of utter joy with my closest friends was enough to make that night unforgettable. What happened next is what burned it into my brain forever.

Pumped up with excitement we decided that it was time for a little chemical relaxation. We called our guy and ordered a forty-dollar bag of weed. We jumped into Jeff's car and drove to our dealer's house to pick it up. Jeff's car was fondly known as the egg. The egg was a 1987

White Subaru GL Hatchback. It fit two comfortably, anything else was a struggle. Some nights, we had as many as twelve people piled in. The rims were spectacular as Jeff would let you know any time you were near his baby, by saying, "them bitches are glowing" or, "them shits is shining". We got our weed and headed down by the water to Shore Road in Bay Ridge to do our thing. It was me, Mikey, Patty and Jeff. Patty rolled it up. We got two monster joints out of the bags and sparked them both. We passed them around between the four of us until there was nothing left. We were high as kites. The music in the car was blasting, and every sound was enhanced tenfold. It was a nice night, and with our senses heightened you could taste the salt in the air from the cool ocean breeze. This was already one of the best nights of our young lives, and we decided to end it right by taking a ride to White Castle in Sunset Park to satisfy our late-night, pot induced munchies. We took the streets, because as high as we were, the speed of the highway was entirely too much to handle. We were driving under the Brooklyn-Queens Expressway, and it was about time for us to turn off and make our way up to Fourth Avenue. Jeff put on his signal and started the process. The only problem was that he picked a block that you weren't allowed to turn on. We were all in our own worlds. I couldn't tell you what we were talking about or if we were talking at all, then, something happened that until this day I can't explain other than divine intervention. Something told me to look to the right, and when I did all I could do was scream. *"LOOK OUT."* Jeff slammed on his brakes and the egg came to an abrupt halt. An eighteen-wheel tractor trailer was exiting the Gowanus expressway, onto Third Avenue, at a high rate of speed. When I looked to my right seconds earlier, all I saw was the headlights, and the huge front grill of the thundering beast. The next few seconds were like slow motion. All I heard was the loud horn, and all I saw was the trailer passing in front of us. It was inches away. The car shook from the force that it produced, and, in that moment, I saw my life flash before my eyes. If I hadn't looked over, we would have surely been dead. The truck never saw us, and never hit his brakes. So many lives would have been altered that night for a bad decision four teenage boys made on an otherwise perfect night. Mikey wouldn't be a father and husband, neither would Jeff. Patty wouldn't be a husband and the best damn DSOA in the DSNY, and I would not be writing this story, with my wife sitting inside, patiently waiting for me to come to bed. I wish I could tell you that was my last brush with death, that I would take that night as a sign of things to come, but I cannot.

Nobody uttered a word the whole ride home. The experience scared the high right out of me. All I could do was stare at the floor and shake. We got to my house, and sat in the living room, that just a few hours before, was the sight of unparalleled exhilaration. Now, a few hours later, we were four scared young boys that couldn't process the enormity of what had just happened. The night would end, and the summer would go on. The Rangers would go on to win the Stanley Cup and the memory of the near-death experience would fade, eventually becoming a joke we would start off with the sentence, *"Hey, remember the night we almost died."* It wasn't a joke, and I don't think any of us really looked at it that way. We were kids and that's how we processed it. That's how we moved on. I would spend the next two months working during the day, playing hockey in the evening and drinking at night. The summer was nearing an end and I couldn't wait to head back up to school and start my sophomore year.

CHAPTER 7

Moving On Up

After an eventful summer back home, it was time to start my sophomore year. Jeff was officially living on campus, so except for the nights he couldn't physically make it to his room, the days of him sleeping on our floor or couch were over. Our second year was much like our first. There was a special every night of the week at the local bars. If we weren't out drinking, we were somewhere on campus, at a party, watching tv or just playing drinking games. Everything, every night, involved alcohol yet I managed to do just enough academically to not get thrown out of school and keep my mother happy. Life at Pace University was like a big party with a twenty-thousand dollar a year cover charge.

During our second semester Ciro started to express interest in becoming an R.A, or Resident Advisor. In layman's terms an R.A was a babysitter for a building full of lunatics. He had been doing it for me and Lou the last two years so why not go a step further and get paid to do it. When I say get paid, I don't mean physically given a paycheck. When you become an R.A, you get your own room with a double bed, and get to live on campus for free. It's a sweet deal if you can handle the responsibility that comes along with the job, and Ciro was nothing if not responsible. With Ciro moving on junior year, I decided to move with Jeff to the upper class-men townhouses that were located up the hill from the regular dorms. Lou would also move there with another one of our fraternity brothers. Little Italy was broken up and while it was the end of an era, we were all happy to be where we were.

The townhouses were great. There were three floors. The main floor had a living room, dining area and full kitchen. The other floors had two bedrooms and a bathroom on each. They usually housed eight guys, but we lived with the RA, so our house was only five. Junior year was much of the same, drinking every night, wherever, and whenever. The thing with the townhouses, is that they were up a hill, far away from the class buildings. There were thirty-five houses. Fraternities, sororities and student athletes comprised most of the population. On any given day, especially in the fall and spring, you could find a barbecue or daytime get together going on. After my disastrous first semester freshman year, I managed to keep my drinking in check just enough to get by. I did everything I could to do as little as possible academically. I only took twelve credits a semester. I never had class on Friday, and any classes I did take were scheduled after four in the afternoon. I figured that by four o'clock I would be able to wake up from my hangover and go to class. Now, separate from the rest of campus, in our own little world, I would rarely make it down that hill. I would spend most afternoons drinking with whoever was around, so even the four o'clock classes became impossible to attend. It was getting in the way of my drinking, so they had to go. I used to say that everybody drank like me. Don't get me wrong, there were a few that did, but more often than not, I was just drifting from house to house, finding people doing what I wanted to do, and that was to get loaded. One night, two friends were arguing. My name came up and one guy said,

> *"You really think Figs is your friend?"*
> *"Figs will be friends with anyone who drinks with him."*

That was another one of those gut punch statements that would become more and more common as my addictions progressed. In that moment, I took offense and harbored a major resentment against the guy who said it. The fact of the matter is he was one hundred percent right. That's why it bothered me so much. My grades took a big hit junior year and this time there was no more hardship grant to fall back on. The only way I would be able to stay at school was to become an R.A. like Ciro. I would just have to raise my GPA slightly to a 2.25 and go through a weekend tryout called RAP weekend. Once again, I did just enough to get by academically. I went to a few classes, wrote a few papers, and sweet talked a few professors to bump me up a half of a grade. Just like that I got a 3.0 that semester. I passed the weekend tryout with flying colors and was hired as an R.A. for my fourth year. I would be returning to the dorm that I spent my first two years in, only this time I would be responsible for maintaining some sort of order in a building full of kids just like myself.

I was always able to make a good first impression. It would be a common theme throughout most of my active addiction. I had the ability to do things well. I had the potential to succeed. My problem was that as soon as I got my foot in the door, my addictions would take over. Drinking or drugging would always become my priority. Once that happened it was only a matter of time before it affected my performance and eventually bled onto everyone around me. It took a while for that to happen as an R.A. Don't get me wrong, I wasn't right for the job from day one. I would drink with my residents. I would never be there when I was supposed to be. The one person I had to write a disciplinary report against was my girlfriend Heather who got alcohol poisoning drinking in my room. The only thing that saved me was my boss. He was a bigger drunk than I was and covering for me kept the heat off him.

I didn't have enough credits to graduate after my "first" senior year so I would have to stay one more year. I would move to the Briarcliff campus which was strictly for housing. I lived in a suite with two of my fraternity brothers. One of those guys was Brinsley, a big, jolly,

Irish kid from Boston. There was nothing not to love about him and we became very close friends. He had a car, so getting to the main campus wasn't a problem. The problem was that he was just as big a drinker as I was. It was a bad combination, and we would spend most days drinking from late afternoon until early morning. We drank in a local bar called Foley's, owned by a local guy named John. He was great guy who took a liking to me the first night we met, and because of that he gave me a job. The best part of that was I would now drink for free. This is when my performance as an R.A. plummeted. I was never on campus. When I was there, I was drunk or sleeping. None of my co workers could depend on me for anything. Their resentment toward me was obvious as well as justified. I was given an ultimatum at the end of the first semester. It was shape up or ship out. By now I lived on campus year-round. My job was there, my girlfriend was there, and I grew to love the area. I considered it home and I wasn't going to get thrown out with four months left to go. My final semester at Pace started in February of 1998. I followed a formula where I did just enough not to get fired as an R.A. and just enough to graduate. I did this all while maintaining my job as a bartender and drinking at an ever-increasing pace.

It was time for graduation and I was so hungover at my ceremony that I had to use my cap as a barf bag. We did the family dinner afterwards and as soon as the family left, I was at Foley's, with Jeff, my girlfriend Heather, and the rest of the townie crew I had become friends with over the last year. Now that school was over it was time to take the real world by storm. At least that's what everybody else wanted me to do. I, on the other hand, was content bartending at Foley's for the foreseeable future as I figured out my next move.

CHAPTER 8

You Bet

Now that school was over, I needed to find a place to live. I could've moved in with Heather, but she was living in Connecticut and I didn't have a car. Getting back and forth to Pleasantville would be too much of a hassle. The university was generous enough to let me stay in the dorms for the summer while I found an apartment. In late June a few of us were hanging out at Foley's drinking and watching baseball. One of my fraternity brothers' parents had an apartment for rent in Montrose, which was about twenty minutes north of Pleasantville. There was a kid Joe looking for a place at the same time as me. Joe went to Pace, but I didn't know him very well. Heather knew him better and assured me that he was a good guy. She was right and me and Joe hit it off the first night we met. We went to look at the apartment, and it was beautiful. It had a brand-new kitchen, a huge dining room, nice size living room and two bedrooms. The price was right, and we decided to take it. We moved in shortly after. Me and Joe had a lot in common. Among our common interests, were a love of sports, and a love of drinking. We spent most of our time at Foley's. If we weren't at Foley's drinking, we were at home drinking. It was a match made in heaven.

It was around this time that I started dabbling in the world of sports betting. There were a few small-time bookies in the area that me, Jeff, Joe, Brinsley, and a few other friends would bet a few games with every week. With my father's history of gambling, and my own addictive tendencies, you'd think I would've stayed away from that life, instead, I dove in headfirst. One afternoon I got a call from my friend's older brother. Jimmy was a connected guy who was always running some sort of scam. His main source of income was a sports book he ran for some local wise guys. His brother told him I was betting with some guys by me, and Jimmy, seeing an opportunity, asked if I wanted to use him instead. When I told him there was a few of us, he made me an offer. If I could get ten guys, he would give me ten percent of whatever the weekly losses were. That sounded good to me. I could get ten guys easy, and I could always use some extra cash. I agreed, and just like that, I became a bookie. Just like that, the words my father said to me shortly before he died were forgotten. Just like that, I was doing exactly what he did.

I developed a solid clientele, consisting of kids from Pace, a few townies, and a bunch of my friends. There was one guy, who generated most of my revenue. His name was Andy. We called him Pipes because of his rock solid forearms. Andy was in his late thirties or early 40's at the time, and made his living working the door at Foleys. He was one of the nicest guys I ever met, but he had a ridiculous gambling habit. It wasn't until much later, that I found out the reason he worked in Foley's, was that he gambled away his tow-truck business years earlier. He started off small, betting a few games a week. He won a few times and lost a few. He always paid on time when he lost, which in the gambling game, builds a trust between bookie and player. As time went on, he began to increase the volume of bets and the amounts on each one. Every time he increased his play, I would have to get the ok from Jimmy before I could put it in. This became a pain in the ass because I had other players. Everything back then was done by phone. Spending a half hour every day on the phone with Andy was bad for business. I asked Jimmy if I could just give Andy the main number, so he could deal with him directly, and iron out any issues they had without me being in the middle. Andy started betting and losing big. One Sunday evening I get a call from Jimmy.

"Tommy, is this fuckin Pipes guy good for this money?" Jimmy questioned.

I had no idea how much Andy was down at this point because he was calling Brooklyn direct.

"Yea Jimmy, why wouldn't he be, he's never been late with a payment since he started with us." I replied.

"I know that, but this fuckin guy is down big, and he's trying to get it all back on tonight's game." Jimmy said with urgency in his voice.

"How big are we talking Jim?" I asked.

"Five thousand big Tommy, I know he's your guy and I trust your judgement, but you gotta tell me right now if he's good for 10 K, if not I can't let him play." Jimmy replied.

Well, that backfired on me. My whole reason for giving Andy direct access was to avoid these situations. Five thousand isn't really that big of a nut in that world, but Andy went from losing hundreds to thousands very quickly and Jimmy was understandably skeptical. Why he waited until it got this far, I have no idea, but now it was on me to figure things out. My next call was to Andy.

"Andy, what the fuck are you doing?" I asked.

"What do ya mean Figgy?" Andy replied like he had no idea what I was talking about.

"Don't treat me like a jerk man. You're down five fuckin thousand in a day and you're trying to double up, you didn't think they were gonna call me and ask if you're good for it?"

"I'm sorry kid, it just got away from me, but I'm good for it, I swear." Andy explained.

"Andy, don't jerk me off. These aren't small time kids like up here. These are serious guys, don't put me in a bad spot."

"Figgy, I would never do that to you, I swear on my kid, I'm good for it."

Andy gave me the gamblers mantra, *I'm good for it.* I know how the gamblers mind works. I grew up in a house with one, and I've been in this same spot myself on one or two occasions. Even if Andy had none of the money to pay us, he would swear on anything and everything he could, including his unborn child, that he would be able to pay. You always think you can win it back, but reality is, most of the time, you don't. The bookie always comes out on top and the house always wins. Against my better judgement I called up Jimmy told him Andy was good. They say there is no such thing as easy money, and they weren't kidding. That night was one of the most stressful of my life. The only way I handled stress was to drink. That night I must've drank thirty beers and a half a bottle of Stoli Orange vodka. The game came down to the final minute and Andy lost. I should've been happy. Instead, I felt like throwing up. There is no way this guy had ten-thousand dollars laying around. He was a doorman at a small Irish bar in Pleasantville, New York. Jimmy felt the same way, and he was up my ass all week.

To both of our surprises, when Thursday came around and I was set to make my collections, Andy came into the bar and handed me an envelope with Ten thousand dollars in clean crisp one hundred-dollar bills. Me and Brinsley drove to Brooklyn and met Jimmy at the Bar up on the Avenue by my mother's house. The Bar was always changing names and owners, but one thing always stayed the same. It was always occupied by wise guys and wannabe wise guys. I handed Jimmy the money, and we had a big toast to our profitable week. He handed me almost two-thousand dollars, which was my cut of my sheet's losses. Andy's nut made up half of that money. Like I said before, there is no such thing as easy money. As quick as it came it was the hardest two grand I ever made, but there was also a strange sense of pride. I was finally in that bar on the corner that my mother always said to stay away from. I was with the older guys from the neighborhood. I was with the guys like my father that I had been trying to be like my whole life. I was adding more and more traits to the character I had been building for years and falling farther away from the person I really was.

Andy would go on to lose a hundred and twenty-seven thousand dollars over the next few months. He always paid on time, and always in clean crisp money. One week, he was down huge. Georgia Tech was playing Syracuse on a Thursday night and Andy had fifteen grand on Georgia Tech. There were guys in the bar that had one, maybe two hundred on Syracuse. He was losing the bet and the guys who had Syracuse were cheering their team on. Andy snapped, and started yelling at one of the guys. I took him into the basement and explained that just because he was out of control, he couldn't be fighting with people who were playing within their means. Andy started weeping like a little child. The stress of the continuous losing finally got to him. Here I am, watching this man cry as he's throwing his life away and all I can see in him was my father's past and my future. I felt guilty, but I told myself he was doing it to himself. If not me, he would be betting with someone else and the money from his losses was supporting my own gambling habit. I felt like a hypocrite, but I took his money anyway. Eventually, his wife would find out that he was draining their life savings and Andy's gambling days were over. Heather, having had enough of me never paying attention to her and my less then legal activities, gave me an ultimatum. It was her, or the life I was leading. I chose the life and that ended our two-year relationship. Whatever little self-control I exhibited for her was now out the window and my lifestyle became wilder than it already was.

The drinking was now an all-day thing. I would start when I woke up and go until I passed out. I also started taking ecstasy on a regular basis and the only time I wasn't under the influence is when I was working at Foleys two nights a week. Any money I was making through taking bets was going right back to Jimmy because I was losing just as much as I was taking in. One Saturday night a bunch of my friends came into the bar after a night out in the city. They wanted to keep the party going up at the townhouses at Pace. I had been drinking and betting baseball all day so I was in no condition to stay up any longer. I asked for some ecstasy, but my guy didn't have any. He reached into his pocket and pulled out a little foil packet about the size of half of my finger. When I asked what it was, he replied, *"It's Larry."* Larry was his code word for cocaine. I had never seen cocaine before and I never thought of doing it myself. He told me it would sober me up and I would be able to party with them some more. I knew that if I did this, I would be crossing a line into a world I knew nothing about. Every ounce of logic and sanity I had left told me not to do it, but as it is with an addict like myself, logic and sanity rarely win out. I took that foil packet into the lady's bathroom. All I knew is what I had seen in movies and on tv. I scooped a small amount onto the top of the toilet tank and made it into a line. I took a twenty-dollar bill out of my pocket and rolled it up. I kneeled over, my head just above the tank, put the twenty to the edge of my nose and snorted it. My nose burned a little and the whole front of my face went numb. I straightened up and snorted what I felt I had left in my nose and that's when it happened. The back of my throat went numb and I felt a surge of energy that I had never felt before. It was like the eight hours of drinking I had just done never happened. I was ready to go for three more days. From that day on I would rarely go a day without cocaine. As soon as I had a certain amount of alcohol in me it was like a switch went off in my brain and I had to have it. I was going through money like it was water.

I even tried selling coke and ecstasy to support my habit. My poor mother worked seven days a week to put me through school and here I was, a bartender, a bookie and a drug dealer. On top of that I was my best customer in all three.

The next year was a haze, fueled by alcohol, cocaine and gambling. I would be up for days at a time, often making late night trips to Mohegan Sun or Foxwoods. There was one trip that stood out from the rest. There was a kid who bartended with me. His name was Matty. Matty was a great dude. He was a baseball player from Pace that I had known for a few years. One night we were counting the register and he somehow lost the quick draw money. It was more than likely thrown away when we cleaned off the bar a half hour before and he was in a full-blown panic. He was on thin ice with John already and he needed to make the quick draw discrepancy right. There was nine hundred dollars in the envelope, and he asked if I could float it to him. I only had three hundred on me and his panic just got worse. He had the bright idea of taking a ride up to Mohegan Sun. Back in the late 90's Mohegan Sun wasn't a hotel yet. The ride sucked, and if you lost, the trip home the next morning was awful. It was two in the morning, and I was in no mood to make the trip. I repeatedly told him that I would talk to John and straighten everything out. He refused to accept any of my reasoning and kept pressing me to take the ride. Eventually I gave in, and we made our way two hours up I-95 to try and win the quick draw money back. I was always up to gamble, but that night I wasn't in the mood. They stop serving alcohol at 2 am, so I really wasn't a happy camper. When we got there, I told him he had two hours to win the money. Either way we were leaving when that time was up. He went to the blackjack tables and I went and played let it ride. After a half hour of sitting with three old ladies blowing smoke in my face, I decided to go sit at a blackjack table. I might as well have some fun. I had three hundred on me, and three hundred wasn't enough to make the ride home all that bad if I lost. It started slow, then the action started to pick up. I started winning a little bit, and then a little more. The game got so fast I blacked out. Anyone who has played blackjack knows that you can win a lot or lose a lot very quickly. The game flies and the decisions are quick. By the time I got up to go to the bathroom I had six thousand eight hundred dollars in front of me. I don't even remember how it happened. I put six thousand in my pocket and put the remaining eight-hundred in the bet circle. Once I lost that eight, I would be done for the night. I never lost the eight. I hit black jack's, I doubled, I split. I did everything right. Matty was at the table directly across from me and noticed the commotion. By now I had twenty people cheering me on. When all was said and done, I walked out with twelve thousand eight hundred dollars. It was thirteen three, but I threw the dealer five hundred for giving me the best cards I've ever gotten in my life. Matty was down a few hundred and he was begging me to stay. I asked him how much he had left. I think it was two hundred. I grabbed his chips, sat at his table, and in three hands won enough for him to replace the quick draw money with nobody being the wiser. I walked out of that place feeling like a gangster, with stacks of cash in each of my inner jacket pockets. The ride home that morning was good and Matty wouldn't stop thanking me when I really should've been thanking him. I keep in touch with him on social media and we talk about that night still today. His name is changed in this story, but you know who you are. That was a night we will never forget my friend.

That was one of the good nights, but there were plenty of bad ones. There were times I had dresser drawers full of money, but there were also times I couldn't pay the rent. I always owed Jimmy money and there were times I was short. When that would happen, I'd send Brinsley to drop the money off or I'd meet one of my other friends and give them the envelope to give to Jimmy. By the time he found out it was short I would be back in Foleys getting hammered and I would ignore his calls. Jimmy was no saint. He took advantage of people on a regular basis to make money, but he had people he had to answer to and I put him in a bad spot many times. He knew me since I was a kid, and I knew he would never hurt me. I took advantage of that and him. He eventually cut me off and my days of being a bookie were over.

The booze and coke filled nights continued and people started noticing my spiral. I looked terrible and acted erratic. John always treated me like a son and he was the first person to sit down with me and voice his concerns. He told me how he saw a lot of his friends mess their lives up with coke. He told me I should cool it. He even offered to send me to rehab if I wanted to go. It meant a lot to me that he cared so much. My father had been gone almost two years now and for the most part he was out of my life long before that. It felt good to have a man in my life to look up to and know that he cared about my well-being. I politely declined his offer and went on partying every night. By now there was no money. Whatever I made at Foleys was going up my nose. I started stealing from the register to support my habit. When I didn't have money for the rent, I would call my Aunt Eileen or borrow money from John to pay it. I would borrow money from John then pay him back with money I stole from his register. How sick is that?

It was May of 2000, and Joe was getting tired of my ways. We barely spoke anymore and I was starting to run out of friends and options, so I did what all good addicts do. I decided it was time for a geographic change. I convinced myself that my problem wasn't the drinking and drugs, it was the lack of structure. I was still living the college life two years after graduating. It was time to go back to Brooklyn and get a real job. My first thought was to become a teacher. I quickly realized that me overseeing children probably wasn't the best fit for me at the time so I called my cousin and asked if there were any openings at the brokerage firm. I worked summers there for six years and now I had the degree needed for a permanent position. She told me there was a spot open in the accounting department and wanted me to go for an interview.

I knew all the people in the firm since I was fifteen years old. They all loved me and thought of me as this cute little kid. The interview was a formality. I spoke to the CFO for about ten minutes and he offered me the job. I was the new clerk in charge of accounts receivable for a multimillion-dollar company and I was to starting the Tuesday after Memorial Day which gave me a week to get my stuff together and move home. I didn't even say goodbye. I left my room a mess with beer bottles full of urine everywhere. When I talked to Joe years later he was happy I was sober. He told me how he wanted to kill me at the time, but knew it wasn't the real me doing those things. He knew the alcohol and coke had a hold of me and partially blamed himself for letting it go on as long as it did. He was in no way to blame and I'm happy I was able to clear the air with him.

I left my family and friends in Brooklyn as a seventeen-year-old kid. Everybody in the firm knew me as that kid. What everyone in Brooklyn and the firm didn't know was what they were getting back was a different person. What they were getting back was an addict and alcoholic with no regard for anyone or anything but himself.

John from Foley's would die tragically four years later just two days shy of his forty-third birthday. He had a massive heart attack while playing hockey. When I found out, I had every intention of going up to Pleasantville for the funeral. An addict always has good intentions, but they just rarely follow through on them. I wound up getting high that day and when my ride called, I didn't answer. A big part of recovery is making amends to the people you harmed along the way. I loved John and wanted to do right by him. Him being gone made that hard to do. As a kid, John had a sister that died of Sudden Infant Death Syndrome. Over the last fifteen years I have donated a small amount from every paycheck to the SIDS Foundation in honor of John. I will continue to do so until I retire. My only hope is that he is looking down proudly at the person I've become.

Rest In Peace.
John Myron
7/2/1961 – 6/30/2004

CHAPTER 9

Homecoming

I was back in Brooklyn, and as much as I loved Westchester, it was good to be home. I would miss the friends I made over the last seven years, but the truth was, most of them were either tired of my nonsense, or moved back home to start their life after college. Jeff and I stayed close and we would visit each other a few times a month. During the last year in Westchester, my life had gotten out of control. The cocaine use made me do a lot of things I wasn't proud of. I told myself the night I got home that I would stop the cocaine, because that was the problem. I was fine when I just drank. Nobody got mad at me, nobody had sit downs with me telling me I needed help when I was just drinking, so that's what I would do. I would only drink and smoke a little weed of course. That was the promise I made to myself.

I got home around five o'clock on Memorial Day. Mom and Aunt Eileen were happy to have me back. They were at my Aunt's house in Pennsylvania for the weekend, but left me a nice dish of chicken parmigiana to welcome me home. I quickly unpacked and called Joey and G to see what they were doing. They were hanging out in G's basement drinking some beers. I ran to the store, grabbed a twelve pack of Corona and headed over. Everybody was happy to see me. We wound up drinking and smoking weed until ten o'clock when I excused myself to go get a good night sleep for my first day of work. It was the first time in a long time that I didn't do any coke and the first time I was able to go to sleep like a normal person in over a year. I had it all figured out now and my life would begin to get back on track. At least that's what I told myself.

I started work the next day and it was like I never left. I was working with the same people in the same building as I did a few years earlier, only now, I was making a lot more money. I started out making thirty-five thousand dollars a year plus a holiday bonus. Forty thousand plus a year and benefits while living at home with the family was a lot of money for me back then. My plan of drinking and smoking weed was going very well and I was going to work every day and learning the job. I said earlier that I always made good first impressions. This was no different. Add to that the fact they knew me already and my cousin had been there since the firm's inception, I could do no wrong. The following Friday I got my paycheck and I was flush with cash. I bought a big bag of weed and headed to G's to start the weekend right. After one hour, two bong sessions and seven or eight Coronas that familiar switch went off in my brain. It was the switch that went off every day for the last year in Westchester. My brain wanted some cocaine. When my brain wanted cocaine, my body would find it. I mentioned my craving to my friends and next thing I knew we had three grams worth of high-quality coke in our hands. I started that night and didn't stop until Sunday afternoon. That's how quick it went right back to the way it was. All it took was one night, and after only two weeks, I was right back to doing the very thing that I had moved back to get away from. Wherever I went, there I was.

As time went on my nights were getting longer. I would leave work at five and get home around six. My Aunt always had dinner ready for me when I got home. She had been semi-retired for a few years and did some medical billing for my mother's boss. She would call me every day around lunchtime and ask me what I wanted for dinner. Whatever I asked her to make was on the table when I got home, no matter what. As soon as I was done eating it was off to the races. It really didn't matter where we were. Whether it was Joey and Patty's house, G's basement, The Bar, Bennet's, or the Monk, there was always a lot of drinking going on and when I was drinking the cocaine was sure to follow. I would be out with the guys until midnight and when they would go home to sleep I would continue the party by myself. I would finish off whatever coke I had left, then desperately try to drink myself to sleep. I was getting two or three hours of sleep a night if I was lucky and it started to catch up with me. One morning I woke up feeling especially awful. I struggled just to get dressed and the train ride was a nightmare. When I got to the office and started to do my morning reports I noticed that my hands were very shaky. I had mornings where I was unsteady, but this was different. My hands shook, and my whole body broke out in a cold sweat. All the color must've drained from my face because a coworker asked if I was ok. I tried getting some fresh air, then went into the bathroom and threw some water on my face. I went outside to have a cigarette and that just made it worse. After an hour of feeling like this I called down to my boss Bart and told him I was feeling sick. I asked if I could take the rest of the day. He came upstairs, took one look at me, and told me to go home. He told me to get some rest and come back in the morning. I took one of the company's taxis home because the thought of getting on a train terrified me at that moment. When I got home my Aunt took one look at me and told me as lovingly as she could that I looked like her mother right before she died. That just made things worse and I was in a full-blown panic. I really felt like I was going to die. I couldn't take it anymore so I took car service down to my mother's office and asked if I could see the doctor.

Dr. Fred was one of my mother's bosses. He is by far one of the best people I've ever known. He had a very calm demeanor and a sick sense of humor. Talking to him was like talking to your father and best friend rolled into one. Even to this day I gravitate towards older men that I can look up to. I was always looking for that father figure and I Found it in him.

"Tommy, what's going on?" Dr. Fred inquired.

"Honestly Doc, I feel like I'm going to die." I said with complete sincerity.

"You're not going to die you asshole." He said jokingly.

He's calling me an asshole for thinking I'm going to die. I'm thinking, if he knew how much coke and booze I shoveled into my body last night, he'd understand where I was coming from.

"Did you drink any alcohol last night?" He asked.

"I had a few beers watching the game." I lied.

"How often do you have a few beers?" He asked.

"A couple of times a week, nothing crazy." I lied again.

"Any drugs Tom?" He asked a little more seriously.

"None." Last lie of the day.

I trusted this man completely, yet when he asked me about my drinking and drug use, I flat out lied to his face. I think he had his suspicions, but knowing me and my mother like he did, he gave me the benefit of the doubt. With the symptoms I presented and my denial of any substance use, he was left with one diagnosis. He told me I had an anxiety attack. He gave me a script for Ativan and said to take one when I got home and any time I felt like this again. I didn't know what Ativan was, but when I got home and took one, I felt better within twenty minutes. The next day I got up and went to work. At five o'clock I felt great so I resumed my normal routine of dinner, drinking and cocaine. The next morning, the death feeling came over me again so I took an Ativan. Like magic, twenty minutes later I felt fine and was able to go to work. This became my new routine and would last for much of the next year and a half.

The rest of 2000 and all of 2001 was much of the same for me. By now I had added Klonipin, Xanax and prescription painkillers to the mix. Most nights consisted of washing down a couple of Percocet or Vicodin with a twelve pack of corona and a little weed. Add some late-night cocaine and a Klonipin or Xanax to stop the shakes and anxiety in the morning and you have yourself a big recipe for disaster. I was struggling to make it to work every day. When I would get there, it was usually late, and it was getting increasingly more difficult to do my job. I would be sitting at my desk on a Friday and look at my computer screen not remembering what I did Monday through Thursday. I was the guy who made sure the firm was getting paid. They would pay the brokers their commission up front. My job was checking our reports against trade tickets for accuracy. The next step was to compare our report with the outside firms, create an invoice and send the bill. Finally, I had to collect. It wasn't like collecting for Jimmy. These brokers were rich for a reason. They were good with money. Two parts of being good with money are to always get paid what you're owed and never paying what you don't. Being in a proverbial blackout and late every day made doing this job close to impossible, so I did what any good addict would do, I made stuff up. I would make up numbers to balance the books. If a company didn't pay us in full, I just lowered the invoice to meet what they paid. I also started taking cabs all over the city and charging to other people's expense accounts because I was trying to play the role of this big shot Wall Street guy. My rationale for this was that they were spending thousands a month on cabs, dinners and drinks. What's another fifty? They'll never miss it. My life was completely out of control and the more I drank, used, lied and manipulated things, the worse it was getting.

CHAPTER 10

Never Forget

It was a Monday morning in early September of 2001. The previous day was spent playing softball in the morning, then watching football and drinking all afternoon. Once nighttime came so did the coke. There I was at four in the morning, wide awake, with only three hours before I had to be up for work. I dozed off for about an hour when my alarm went off. I was a mess. The shakes were there, the cold sweat too. I was in such a rush to get out of the house that I forgot to take my pill. By the time I realized that I didn't have them on me it was too late. I was on the train going over the Manhattan Bridge and I wasn't doing well at all. I showed up at the office a half hour late as usual and sat at my desk. I didn't even turn the computer on. There was no way I was making it through the day. I didn't even tell anyone I was leaving. I just called a cab and went home. I called Bart when I was on the road already. By now he was used to my act. If it weren't for my cousin and my past relationship with the firm, I would've been fired a long time ago. He just told me to get some rest and report to his office the next day for his run of the mill get your shit together speech. As soon as I got home I took a Klonipin, a Xanax and settled into the recliner in my basement. I was out cold within a half hour. I woke up around three in the afternoon and just watched movies the rest of the day. I was so exhausted that I didn't even go drinking that night, which was a first for me. I woke up early the next day feeling refreshed. It was gorgeous out. As I boarded the train to work, I was dreading the lecture I was about to get. By now I knew exactly what to say to escape with yet another warning. That lecture wasn't meant to be that day. I said earlier that some events are burned into your memory forever. What happened that day was not only burned into my memory, but the memory of millions. It would change everything. It would change our city, our country and the entire world as we knew it.

I worked in Midtown on Forty Third Street and Madison Avenue. I hated crowded trains so if I had the time to spare, I would take the local train and transfer downtown at Chambers Street to one of the numbered trains. I believe it was the 6 train. When I did this, I would always get a seat and it would leave me off in Grand Central Station right outside of my building. When I got to my office, I decided to go to my floor first and get a cup of coffee before I went to see my boss. When I arrived, I was met with questions from my coworkers.

"Did you hear what happened?" One of them asked.

I thought they were asking me what happened the day before that caused me to disappear with no warning. I offered up some lame excuse about a stomach issue.

"No Tommy, we said did you hear what happened?"
"No. What happened?" I replied.

I was fully expecting them to tell me someone had caught on to my less than accurate bookkeeping. What came next was something completely different.

"A plane hit the World Trade Center." One of them said with a sense of shock in his voice.
"What?" I shot back.

My first thought was some maniac was trying to hang glide from one building to another, or a small plane with an inexperienced pilot went off course and crashed into the building. These were both awful things, but not the scope of what actually happened. As we were talking another plane hit the second tower. It was becoming evident that this was more than some accident. The news channels started to scramble, and reports were coming from every direction. A few of us walked down to Fifth Avenue. From there you had a clear view of the towers, even from twelve miles away. What we saw was something beyond our comprehension. A jet plane was sticking out of the side of the tower, black smoke and fire engulfed the air around it. We ran back to the office and started making calls. Patty was with the Sanitation Department for about a year at this point and worked at Manhattan 4 Garage, located on the West Side Highway. He had a better view of what was going on and his exact words to me were to get out of dodge. As we were all trying to process what was going on, news reports of a plane hitting the Pentagon came flooding in. It was clear to everybody that we were under attack. I turned to Bart and said,

"You can fire me if you want to, but I'm getting the fuck out of here right now."

At this point survival instinct starts to kick in. Even though I was a safe distance away from the Trade Center, I didn't know what was coming next. What if it was Grand Central? I bolted out of the office and started to walk. The thing is, there was nowhere to go. No trains were running, and all the bridges and tunnels were shut down. You feel alone in moments like these, almost like you're in a tunnel. You can't hear anyone or anything around you. Just then I heard a noise. It was a voice.

"Figs, Figs, Figs, YO FIGS!"

I came out of my daze and my friend Frankie was standing in front of me. Frankie was a guy from Brooklyn that I met in Pace. We became pretty good friends in Westchester, mainly because of our mutual interest in cocaine. The last thing I needed at that point was cocaine, but I did need a friend. Frankie was that friend and we began our journey back to Brooklyn.

After talking about our limited options, we decided that we were going to walk home from Midtown Manhattan. That sounds crazy, but it was our only choice. We started to make our way downtown. We made a stop to pick up Frankie's sister at her office on 23rd Street, then we headed to Frankie's girlfriend's apartment to grab something quick to eat. There had been buzz in the streets that the towers had fallen. We thought to ourselves there was no way those buildings came down. Sure enough, by the time we got to his girlfriends and put on the news, the twin towers had indeed collapsed. I needed a drink. It had been two days since my last one and I didn't take any Xanax or Klonipin that morning. This whole day was insane and my nerves were shot. I downed a few beers, ate a slice of pizza, and we continued our mission. As we got further downtown the already somber mood of the city got even worse. People were walking around like zombies. If you've ever been to Manhattan you know that there is always a buzz. Everyone is moving to get where they must go at a rapid pace. On this day it was different. The enormity of what happened seemed to paralyze everybody and there was more of a deliberate feel to people's movements. It wasn't slow by any means, but it wasn't fast. The city was in shock.

As we made our way around ground zero, we were directed towards the Brooklyn Bridge. The air was heavy and suffocating. The smell was unforgettable and something I can't put into words. As I got halfway over the bridge I stopped and looked back towards Manhattan. The island we just left was unrecognizable, clouded by black smoke. There were so many thoughts running through my head. Thousands of people got up that day, went to work just like I did, and were never coming home. Their families would be destroyed. Children were orphaned. Parents would have to bury their kids. Husbands and wives were widowed. It hit me in that moment that this was so much bigger than anything I had ever witnessed.

We would make it to Frankie's house in downtown Brooklyn. We were covered in the gray dust that would inhabit the city for weeks and months to come. Frankie drove me home and I was greeted by G and the two Joeys' with a big hug. I went and hugged my aunt and mother. I went to my room and decompressed. I took a long hot shower and laid in my bed for at least an hour just staring at the ceiling. My Aunt made my favorite cheese and parsley sausage wheel for dinner. Joey and G ate with me. I was on auto pilot and what I did next was what I'd been doing every night for a long time. I went upstairs and took a bunch of Percocet from my aunt's drawer. We went and bought a case of Michelob bottles and got drunk and high. I used this day as an excuse to get high for a long time. So many people's lives were broken in ways that could never be fixed and here I was making it about myself. I was a selfish, self-centered drug addict and my life would get much worse before it ever got better.

I would later find out that five people I knew died in those buildings. They weren't close friends, but they were part of my life at one time or another. I knew and liked them all. I went to high school and hung out in the Annex with three of them. I played hockey with two of those three. The fourth was a customer and friendly acquaintance from Foleys. He started working at Cantor Fitzgerald two years earlier to make a better life for his family. The fifth was the father of one of my Fraternity brothers. I had met him only a couple of times. He was a true gentleman and raised two fine sons. He died helping others live and the Hold the Door Foundation was started by his son in his honor.

Rest In Peace.
Richie, Rob, Jude, Pauly, Ronald and the rest of the 2,996 that lost their lives that day and the thousands more who have lost their lives since due to 9-11 related illnesses.
9/11/2001
WE WILL NEVER FORGET!

CHAPTER 11

Show Me The Money

The days, weeks, and months following 9/11 were some of the most pivotal moments in our country's history. We were attacked on our own soil, and the sense of security we had all come to know turned into a feeling of vulnerability and fear. We would declare war on our enemies, and the uncertainty of what the future would hold weighed on the hearts and minds of many. You couldn't turn on the television or open a newspaper without seeing the horrifying images of that day, and at any given moment you could find coverage of a funeral service on your local news broadcast. It was much of the same in the neighborhood. It seemed like there was a service every day at the local church or funeral home. I attended wakes and masses for the guys I went to school with and the hurt in the faces of their families is something I will never forget. As for me, not much had changed. My drinking and drug use were getting worse, and my performance at the firm was at an all-time low. Things were about to come to a head in more ways than one.

One Monday morning I was called in to Bart's office around 10 a.m. He was concerned about my performance and often disheveled appearance and asked me what was going on. Being the manipulative addict I was, I told him the reason for this was that I had been attending services for friends who died in the towers for weeks and hadn't been getting any sleep. I poured it on thick, and by the end of the conversation I was given a two-month paid leave of absence. They knew I was having problems long before that day. They knew I was on anxiety medication, and I'm sure they knew I had issues with alcohol and drugs. They were giving me an opportunity to get help and come back with a clean slate. I thanked him and left the office for what was supposed to be the start of my healing process. Walking out that door I had every intention of getting the help they were suggesting, but once again an addict's good intentions are rarely followed through.

I would spend the next two months going to therapy during the day to appease my family and show the firm I was doing something to help myself. As soon as I would leave my counselors office I would go home and grab a few Percocet from my aunt's drawer. Once those kicked in, I'd grab a twelve pack and go to Joey's or G's and smoke some weed. I would then go to The Bar or Bennet's to drink for a few more hours. By the end of the night, without fail, I would be in my house, by myself, with a bag of coke, another six pack, and a few Klonipin or Xanax to put myself to sleep. When December rolled around, and it was time to go back to work, I was more of a mess than I was when I left.

They tried everything. They changed my hours from nine to five to nine-thirty to five-thirty. They even tried giving me more responsibility. The accounts payable clerk was leaving the firm so instead of hiring someone else to take her place, they would give me her job on top of my own. If I did well, I would get a ten-thousand dollar raise. Of course, I accepted. A raise sounded good to me, but I couldn't even do my own job and now I was taking on another. With more responsibility came more stress, and with more stress came more drinking and drugs. It all came to a head in January of 2002. My accounts receivables were a disaster so I started to go to the brokers to see if they could get the money we were owed from their trades. I remember one female broker trying her best to help but giving up after she realized the mess that I had created. It felt like the world was crashing down on my shoulders. I couldn't tell anyone what I had been doing. Every report I had created the last year and a half was tainted. The firm's credibility would be destroyed, Bart would lose his job, my cousin's reputation would be forever tarnished, and I could very likely be brought up on charges and go to prison. I kept drinking and drugging to forget the situation I was in, but it wasn't working. Finally, I snapped. I stormed into Bart's office one morning screaming that I wasn't appreciated and demanding my ten-thousand dollar raise. That's right. I was creating fake reports for a year and a half. I was taking company cars everywhere and charging other people. I was never on time. I never stayed late. I left work three or four times a month because I partied too much the night before and couldn't take the withdrawals. When I was there, I was usually in a benzo induced blackout. When they paid me for two months to stay home and get some help all I did was get worse. I do one month of accounts payable and there I was, in Bart's office, like I was the best thing on Wall Street since Gordon Gecko. That's how sick I was. In that moment I believed everything I was saying to him. After I was done with my tirade, he just looked at me and said,

"Tommy, are you fucking kidding me?"

I hated that response at the time. Looking back on that day, if it were me, and I had some kid screaming at me like that after all I did to help him, my words wouldn't have been as nice.

"I'm done, I fucking quit." I yelled as I stormed out of his office.

Just like that I was done. All the chances they gave meant nothing to me. My cousin putting herself out there for me meant nothing. The four accountants I worked with daily who stuck up for me when I didn't deserve it meant nothing. The people whose careers I put in jeopardy meant nothing. The only thing that mattered to me was self-preservation. I thought if I got out of there, they'd just forget about me. We could all move on with no one being the wiser. I couldn't be more wrong. I left a mess and that mess had to be cleaned up. It was one thing having ten different reports a month when I was the only one looking at them. It's another thing when someone else goes in there and investigates. They found everything. They found all the false reports. They found the invoices for the cab rides and figured out how I had been writing them off to other people's expense accounts. Bart called me every day for weeks demanding that I come to the office and answer for what I had done, even threatening to involve the federal authorities. I refused, eventually avoiding his calls. My cousin was mortified. I don't think she looked at me for three years after that and we lived in the same house. When all was said and done, the fact that I didn't steal any money boded well for me. They wouldn't press charges, but there were stipulations. They wanted me to pay for the cabs. I don't remember the exact amount, but it was a few thousand dollars. I never paid them back. My cousin did. I wasn't allowed to enter the building I worked at ever again and I was never to apply for a job anywhere in the Wall Street community. I should've been ashamed of what I had done, but I wasn't. The truth is, I was relieved it was over and I got out unscathed. It was a month-long process, and everybody involved was put under a tremendous amount of stress. The whole situation was another one that I should've learned from. The cause and effect of everything that happened at the firm were a direct result of alcohol and drugs. I should've stepped back and taken and honest look at where my life was heading. Instead, I was in The Bar, Bennet's and G's basement, drinking, getting high, and trying to forget.

CHAPTER 12

PSYCH-OUT

It was now February 2002. The aftermath of what happened at the firm was still fresh in everybody's mind. My family and friends were concerned about me. I was sleeping all day and drinking and getting high all night. With no money coming in, and pressure mounting from family and friends, I decided it was time to take a break. I knew my drug use was out of control, and if I could just stop using, maybe I could get my life together. One night, drunk and high, I wrote a letter to my mother and aunt. It read like this.

Mom and Aunt, please read this together, and I'll talk to you about it when I get up.

Love T.

Hi Guys,
Before I start, I want none of you to blame yourselves for this because there is only one person to blame, and that is me. For a few years I've been lying to myself about a problem I have. I thought I could beat it by myself, but I was wrong, and now it's getting to the point where I know I need help. I know it's impossible for you not to think less of me, because I think less of myself. I don't know how it happened, but it did. I'm not a bad person and I never wanted this to happen, but it did and now I have to get help for it. Some things are easier than others. The gambling was

easy for me to stop. This is too hard, and no matter how long I stay away, I always go back. It has a lot to do with the anxiety and moods I get in, and I don't want to live like this anymore. I can see my friends getting concerned, and before it gets completely out of control, I need to stop it. I don't want to die, and I don't want to punish myself anymore for things I had or have no control over. I love all of you so much, and I know this will probably hurt you just as much as me, but you are the only ones I can come to because I'm finally admitting I have a problem. I'm sick and I need help, please help me find the help I need. I love you. T

My mother saved that note and gave it to me about three months before I started writing this book. Even now, I can feel the pain that I was in. Everything I wrote in that letter was from the heart. I knew I had a problem, and I had every intention of trying to fix it. Once again, an addict's best intentions are rarely followed through.

When I woke up the next day, my mother and aunt were waiting for me upstairs. They were sad and disappointed, but they were also relieved and optimistic. Their little boy was finally going to get the help he needed. They were more than willing to help and they got on the phone with Dr. Fred. After numerous calls back and forth, we settled on North Shore Hospital in Long Island. I was told they had a drug and alcohol program there and it was close to Dr. Fred's house. Knowing he was close by made me feel more at ease about the whole thing. It was Friday night, and a bed was opening on Monday. That left me two days to prepare. I prepared by watching Team USA Olympic hockey, drinking forties, eating Percocet, and sniffing coke. I figured why not get it all out of my system. One last run before my life would change for the better. Sunday night came, and I said goodbye to my friends. We drank some beer, smoked some weed, and gave each other hugs. They wished me well, and I was off.

I woke up on Monday morning and I was nervous. I didn't know anything about what I was getting into. My only references were tv shows and movies, where a character would go to rehab and come back a new person, so that's what I made up my mind to expect. I needed to take the edge off so I took a few Klonipin. The edge was still there so I took a few more. By the time I got the edge off I had taken twenty-one milligrams. That is a lot of Klonipin. I slept the whole ride there and when I woke up Dr. Fred was standing outside my aunt's car looking at me through the window. I got out of the car, still very much sedated from the pills as we walked to the emergency room entrance together. They did a battery of tests on me and asked me a lot of questions. I was very honest with all my answers and it was decided that I needed to be monitored for a few hours before they made any decisions about the care I was to receive. One doctor said to me,

"Thomas, your brain is like a gas tank. The chemicals in your brain are the fuel to your body. When you take all these drugs, you use all the gas. When your body tries to go, there's no gas left, and that's why you feel the way you do."

I had a massive amount of Klonipin in my system and I was overwhelmed by the whole situation, so the gas tank analogy made no sense to me in that moment. Many years later I know exactly what he was talking about.

After five or six hours, the doctor came to see me. He said I would be going upstairs to start my stay. I was happy to hear the news because I couldn't watch my mother cry anymore and the Klonipin was wearing off, so my anxiety about the whole thing was starting to ramp up. If I had more time to think I might have run the other way. I don't remember what floor it was, but when we got out of the elevator it wasn't what I was expecting. When you see rehab in the movies it's usually this beautiful place with big green trees and a clear blue pool. People are playing cards and ping pong, talking about what their plans are when they get out to start their new lives. That isn't what this was. When the doors opened there was a large steel door about fifty feet from the elevator. The doctor rang a bell and a buzzer sounded. He opened the door and we walked inside. It was dark and uninviting. It smelled like sick people. There were no games, no pool and no trees. The mirrors weren't even glass. They were a blurry tin looking material that you often see in shows about prison. We walked up to the desk and the man behind asked me for my belt and shoelaces. He gave me hospital issued slippers which were not much more than socks with some rubber on the bottom. I turned to Dr. Fred with a confused look on my face. He looked at me with the eyes of a sad puppy and said,

> *"Tommy, this is the Psychiatric unit of the hospital, you're going to be spending the next couple of weeks here."*

Whoa, wait a minute. I thought I was going to rehab. I thought I was going to learn how to stop using so much cocaine. You people are sticking me in the nut house. I was livid. I looked at my mother and my aunt. I was waiting for them to save me. I was waiting for them to say this isn't for you. I was waiting for them to say let's go home and figure this out. What I saw were two women who didn't know what to do with the boy they raised. I saw hurt in their faces. I could feel their desperation when I looked in their tear-filled eyes. In that moment, when I realized that nobody was coming to save me, I broke down in tears. How did it get to this? How did my life get so out of control that I wound up in this place? I didn't want to stay. I begged them to take me home, but they couldn't. The doctor in the ER with the gas tank analogy, was a psychiatrist. The answers I gave him in my intake interview, his consultation with Dr. Fred, and the amount of alcohol and drugs in my system, led them to believe that the safest place for me was there, in the psych ward, under medical and psychological supervision for the foreseeable future. I hugged my aunt and mother tight. When I told them I was sorry, my mother couldn't take it anymore and walked away weeping loudly. My aunt, always the calming voice in my life, looked me in the eyes, with her hands cradling my face she told me she loved me, and that she would see me soon. She walked to my mother who was standing by the big steel door, the buzzer sounded, the door opened, and they left. I was alone and scared, not knowing what was going to happen next.

I quickly got on the phone and called my best friends Joey and Patty, telling them where I was and how they had to get me out. I told them everybody there was crazy. I told them about the guy that was walking around with no shirt on yelling at the walls and the chairs, and the old lady who just sat in the corner mumbling obscenities to herself. I even cried to their mother, who had always been there for me when I was struggling. I was telling anybody who would listen that I didn't belong where I was. Apparently, I was the only one who believed what I was saying. They all just told me to get better, and they'd be there when I got home. After exhausting all my options, I had to come to terms with the fact that maybe this is where I belonged. It was going to be my home for a little while so I better get with the program. I was given a buddy, someone who has been at an institution for a while, to show me around and make the first day a little easier. My buddy was a guy named Ulysses. Ulysses was a forty-something year old black man form North Carolina. He told me that every time he came up north to see his girlfriend he wound up in jail or a psych ward. He was a nice guy, and I felt comfortable with him right away. He told me who to talk to and who not to. He told me who the drug and alcohol people were, and he told me who was there for straight mental illness. He happened to be both. He told me how to get hot dogs and hamburgers for lunch and dinner instead of the bland hospital food that was normally served. The most important thing he told me is to go along with the program and not to cause any problems. If I did that, he said I would be out in no time. Ulysses showed me to my room and told me he would catch up with me later that night. Ulysses acted up shortly after that and was given a powerful sedative that caused him to sit silently and drool on himself for the next few days. He was eventually transferred to another facility and I never saw him again.

As I started to unpack, the feelings of guilt and shame overwhelmed me. I couldn't control the tears and I cried for a half hour straight. How did I get here? I was given every opportunity in life. I had all the potential in the world. I was twenty-six years old. I had a college degree. This wasn't supposed to happen to me. The noise in my head was deafening. Just then a nurse knocked on my door. She told me that if I was interested, there was a twelve-step meeting down the hall for people who have a problem with alcohol. I politely said that I wasn't there for alcohol, I was there for cocaine, and I didn't think I needed to sit in on that meeting. She suggested I check it out anyway. She said that I may hear something that could help me. Considering I had nothing else to do, and the more time I spent in my own head the worse I felt, I decided to check it out. A man in his mid-forties led the meeting. He made the trip from Staten Island to share his story with us. As he was speaking all I could think to myself is what kind of loser drives all the way here from Staten Island to talk to a bunch of mental patients. The more he spoke though, the more I was interested. He told his story with such honesty. It was hard not to feel the emotion he was giving off. He said that at his worst he would drive form Staten Island to East New York, Brooklyn to buy crack. He would spend all his money on the drugs and had to go through people's garbage to find cans that he would return for the five-cent deposit to have enough money to get home. His story was moving and even brought a few patients to tears. Unfortunately, once I heard the word crack, everything he said after that went in one ear and out the other. I compared my story to his and didn't hear the message of hope that he was trying to get across. When it came time for me to share, I opened by saying that I was not an alcoholic. I said I did too much cocaine and my life got out of control, but I was twenty-six with a college degree. I can go out and have a few beers with my friends while watching a game and everything would be fine. I will never get to the point of smoking crack or collecting cans in the street. An hour before this, I was standing by myself in a dark room crying like a little baby over the mess my life had become. Now I'm sitting in a twelve step meeting, in a psych ward, telling the guy who has been there, done that and come out the other end, that I was better than him. He pulled me aside after the meeting and told me that if I kept thinking the way I was thinking that I would keep doing the things I was doing. He told me that crack was a yet for me and if I didn't take an honest look at my situation, everything that happened to him was a real possibility for me. He hugged me and told me he would pray for me. He handed me a blue book that looked like a bible and told me I should read it. I thanked him and went back to my room. I put the book in my suitcase, got my anti-seizure and comfort meds and went to sleep.

After a few days the shakiness started to subside and the cobwebs in my brain started to clear. I was going to groups and individual counseling every day. I figured out exactly what they wanted to hear and I told them. I took Ulysses advice and just went with the program. I was notified by my counselor that I would be going home in the exact two-week time frame originally stated. When my mother and aunt came to visit, they couldn't get over how good I looked. I was eating three times a day. I was getting seven hours of sleep every night, and most importantly it was the first time in ten years that I went more than a day or two without any alcohol or drugs in my system. I can honestly say it was the best I felt in a long time, and I was excited to go home and get a fresh start.

The morning I was set to leave the counselors and my fellow patients threw a small going away breakfast for me. It felt good to feel loved and wanted. I had been so messed up for so long, that I had lost all of self-esteem and self-worth. The patients and counselors in that place gave me a small glimpse of what it was like to have that back. My words to the group were that I loved them all, but I hope I never saw any of them again. My aunt was coming to pick me up. When the buzzer sounded and the door was opened for me to leave, my counselor said to me,

> *"Remember what that guy told you the first night here. If you keep thinking the way you think, you'll keep doing the things you do. Take what you learned here and apply it out there. I never want to see you in this place again Tommy. Best of luck to you. God Bless."*

Those words meant a lot to me. I told the intake desk to keep my Klonipin because I didn't need them anymore. I was ready to give this an honest try. My aunt picked me up and even let me drive her car home. It felt good to be trusted. It felt good to be alive. I was going to start a six-month outpatient program the next day and I had the twelve step meeting lists for Brooklyn in my bag. I got home, unpacked, sat on my bed and looked in the mirror. For the first time in a long time I really saw myself and I had no idea who I was. I had no idea how to live without drugs and alcohol. I had every intention of going to a meeting that night. Once again, my intentions and my addict brain weren't on the same page. Just ten hours after being released I was drinking with my friends. I never gave myself a chance. A few days later, at a house in Hunter Mountain that my friends rented for the winter, that familiar switch went off in my head, and I was back doing cocaine. I failed three urine tests in two weeks at the outpatient program and was asked to leave. Four weeks earlier, I told the guy who spoke that first night in psych, that I didn't have a problem with alcohol. I told him I'd never be like him. Four weeks later, I was back doing what I was doing because I never stopped thinking how I was thinking. I forgot the pain I was in. I forgot the feelings of guilt and shame. I forgot about the noise that dominated my thoughts that first night in the hospital. I forgot everything they told me and I was off to the races.

CHAPTER 13

Oxymoron

The day I was being released from the hospital, I sat in the processing room while I waited for my Aunt to pick me up. I met a kid named Mike who was coming in as I was going out. Mike was in his early twenties, but he looked like an old man that hadn't eaten in days. The skin around his eyes was dark, and he had a blank stare that lacked emotion. We started talking about why we were there. I told him my story and he told me his. He had been arrested a week before on possession of a controlled substance. The drug he was in possession of was Oxycontin. I had seen them in my aunt's drawer when I would take her Percocet, but I never knew what they were. He went on to tell me that Oxycontin was a time released form of oxycodone, the opiate found in Percocet. He told me he had been snorting and smoking them for a year and was completely strung out. He detoxed in jail, and when he got out, immediately started using again. His family brought him there, because just like mine, they didn't know what else to do. I wished him well and went on my way.

After the first outpatient incident, I went on to get thrown out of three more for giving dirty urines. I was back to doing nothing during the day and partying at night. The counselors in the hospital would tell me easy does it and one day at a time. Those words mean a great deal to me today, but back then they were just an excuse to avoid responsibility. Any time my family or friends pressed me about my plans going forward I would throw those words in their face. I would tell them that I was sick and this is what they told me to do. They also told me to not drink and drug, go to outpatient, counseling and to attend a twelve-step program regularly. Easy does it seemed to fit my schedule much better. One day while I was home alone, I decided to grab a few Percocet from my aunt. I went up to her apartment and took my usual handful. As I was closing the drawer, I noticed the bottle of Oxycontin. I remembered the conversation with Mike in the hospital. I decided to take a few. By a few, I mean twenty. They were eighty milligrams each. Twenty would set me up for a month. My aunt started to notice her Percocet missing and I was the usual suspect. By doing this I figured it would calm the heat down. I put them in a little glass jar and hid them in a pair of socks in the top drawer of my dresser. In my heart I knew I shouldn't take one. As insane as my addict mind was there was a glimmer of common sense that screamed DANGER every time I contemplated the thought.

A few weeks later, on an early spring Saturday afternoon we decided that we were all going to go out in Bay Ridge. The Wicked Monk was the choice and we started pre-gaming right after lunch. By the time nine o'clock came I was knee deep in the bag. The switch in my head was going off again and I got myself a couple of grams of cocaine for the night. I snorted a few lines before we left the house and I was ready to go. The Monk always had a nice crowd on Saturdays and this night was no different. We drank and listened to a band until one in the morning. I would go to the bathroom every half hour to do a line or two. Like most nights out we decided to finish up at The Bar with a few friends that worked at the local catering hall. By now I must have been twenty-five beers deep between home and the Monk. The coke was keeping me going, but it was running out. At that point I remembered the Oxycontin I had slipped in my pocket before I left the house. The DANGER buzzer was going off in my head and even a head full of cocaine and corona knew this was a bad idea. Eighty milligrams is way too much Oxy. Instead of listening to the warnings in my head I decided that if eighty was too much, forty would be something I could handle. I broke the little green pill in half, flipped it in my mouth and chased it down with another Corona. As I'm writing this I just imagine toilet flushing sounds, because that's exactly what that half of a pill started. What I didn't remember is that there was a time released coating on it. The reason Mike was sniffing and smoking them is because breaking the seal made it all hit you at once. Hit me all at once is exactly what the forty milligrams did. I vividly remember standing at the bar, my left arm around Patty's shoulder as he was picking songs from the jukebox. A warm feeling started rising from my feet all the way up to my face. I had taken many Percocet and Vicodin up to that point, but this was a much more powerful rush. By the time it ran its course up into my head I felt like I was in my own little world. I told Patty that this was the best I ever felt in my life. The rush was so strong that I got violently sick, throwing up three times. The more I threw up, the stronger the feeling of euphoria became. I felt like I was floating. I felt like nobody could touch me. I felt at peace for the first time in years. This was the feeling I had unconsciously been searching for my whole life. I didn't care who was around me. I didn't care what anybody thought. This is how I wanted to feel forever. A choice was made that night that started an obsession and because of that obsession my life would become a much darker place. Little did I know that a conversation in a hospital and a little green pill would alter the course of my life for years to come.

CHAPTER 14

Like a Toy Soldier

The summer of 2002 was when the wheels started to fall off. It had been five months since I got out of the hospital, and I was going harder than ever. Drinking a case of beer and smoking three or four blunts a day was normal. Painkillers and cocaine were added to the mix three or four times a week depending on my ability to get my hands on money or the drugs themselves. I had been talking to a girl that I went to Pace with. Her name was Linda. We started as friends but there was always something more there. She had the same fondness for getting high that I did, and I think that fueled our feelings for each other. She was a beautiful and sweet girl and we always had fun together but something always got in the way of us taking it to another level. We would go to Brinsley's house in Boston every summer for a huge house party. All my friends from Brooklyn and all my friends from college in one place. Add in Brinsley and his brother's friends from Massachusetts and their family and you had one hell of a three-day long party. Much like the summers past me and Linda wound up hanging out together, mostly just drinking, eating pills, sniffing coke and making out. The crazy thing about addiction is that even in a room full of people you can feel so alone. Maybe the feelings were real, maybe they weren't. All I know is that when we were together, I didn't feel alone and maybe she didn't either. Maybe that's why we were drawn to each other. Maybe we were just two broken people looking for something to make us feel whole. Whatever it was, it felt right, and it felt good. I wanted more out of it and by the end of that weekend I think she did too.

The next weekend was our annual block party in Brooklyn. All the same crew from Boston only now in Brooklyn, insanity being the only word I can use to describe it. Linda had agreed to come this year. I invited her a few times before, but this was the first time she said yes. G was seeing her friend Marie so that probably made it easier for her to come. Whatever got her there, I was happy she came. Most people get deserts brought to parties they host. Some people get cookies. Some get a case or two of beer. Not for my parties. For me, they brought a bottle of Percocet. I was six months out of a psych ward for alcohol and drug use and now I have people bringing me painkillers as a gift. Of course, I accepted their gift and instead of spreading the wealth, I took the whole bottle myself. Like it was a bag of skittles I swallowed twenty 10 milligram Percocet at once. I washed down with a Corona and that was just the beginning of a crazy day ahead.

It was a day of more. More alcohol, more cocaine, more pills, more weed, more ecstasy and more insanity. Me and Linda were getting along great. It's kind of hard not to get along with all the shit we had flowing through our systems. Just as I thought to myself this relationship was finally going to the next level a tornado would swoop into my life. Her name was Gina. She was five years younger than me and I hadn't seen her since she dated my friend Joey back in the day. Her cousin lived on my block and she was there for the party. When you're eighteen and thirteen you don't look at a girl in that way. She's a little kid at that point. She was twenty-one years old now and she had really grown into a beautiful young woman. She came over and said hello and gave me a big hug. Throughout the night I noticed her looking in my direction a few times but never thought anything of it. Finally, her aunt told me that she has had a crush on me since she was a little girl and heard I moved back to Brooklyn a couple of years earlier. She had recently broken up with her boyfriend and came to the block party to specifically see me. I was flattered and very interested. There was only one problem. I was there with Linda. As the night started to wind down, me and Linda went back to my house. We messed around for a little while, but the booze and pills got the better of her and she fell asleep. I had been doing bumps of cocaine all day so I was still up for a party. I knew there were still people outside, so I went back down to Patty's house. When I got down the block Gina was there. With Linda back at my house she was very flirtatious. We played some drinking games with my friends, but it wasn't long before we were off by ourselves making out. I had kissed a lot of girls up to that point of my life, but this was different. It was almost like the first Oxycontin I took. I was hooked and I wanted to feel that way all the time. I had the decency to cut it short that night, but it was a force of its own. Linda left my house at one o'clock the next day and I was on the phone with Gina five minutes later. I asked her to come over later that night to "watch a movie". She agreed and I couldn't wait. The only problem was that I felt like I was going to die. Between the coke, Percs, ecstasy, weed and alcohol the night before, my body felt like it was going to shut down. I needed quick relief and I thought "hair of the dog". I went upstairs and got some Oxycontin. I had been laying off them for a while, trying to stick to regular Percs, but I needed something strong and quick. I chewed one 80, swallowed another, and started drinking some Coronas. Within five minutes the one I chewed made me feel normal again. A half hour later the one I swallowed kicked in and I felt nice. By the time she got there I was feeling no pain at all. We spent the night together and had a great time. We didn't have sex. We just kissed and messed around but that instant obsession I felt the night before was there. It was like someone lit a fire in me. She was the final ingredient to my cocktail. I was so lost in my addiction that I couldn't see it for what it was. Like most addicts I try to fix inside problems with outside solutions. The alcohol and drugs worked for a long time, but now it was getting to the point of them making everything worse.

The worse I felt the more I did. I thought if I could find a good girl and get a good job everything would get better. The thing I didn't realize was the problem was within myself and no outside material, human, or chemical solution was going to solve that. I spent the last year trying to get Linda to get more serious and the minute she lets her guard down I do to her the very thing she was trying to avoid. She was supposed to come down later that week. I called her and told her what happened the night of the party and that I didn't think we should see each other anymore. It truly wasn't my intention to hurt her but once again an addict's intentions and the reality of their actions rarely mesh. With the flick of a switch my human drug of choice changed from Linda to Gina. I should've seen it for what it was, a girl's childhood crush and a recent breakup. All my friends warned me that it had rebound written all over it. They warned her about my tendency to drink and get high all day every day. They knew where it was going to end up and they knew one or both of us would be hurt, but the physical connection coupled with both of our needs for something good in our lives was too strong and neither one of us listened. The fact that everybody was against it made it even better.

Gina lived in Long Island and I didn't have a car so the only way we would see each other is if she came to Brooklyn. One or two nights a week she would drive in after work and sleep over, then do the same on Friday and stay until Sunday. Even I was shocked by her motivation and excitement about the whole thing. I had nothing going for me and wasn't even trying to get myself right, but I stopped questioning it and just went with the flow. She was beautiful, fun to be around and at that point she was the only positive thing in my life. When I was with her all the noise in my head went away. Her cousin told her I was a junkie and a drunk and she didn't care. She was all in on me and that made me feel good. Maybe this is what I needed all along, a girl who would support me no matter what. We talked about our future. My plan was to take the test for the NYPD, become a cop and get stationed in Queens. We would move in together and I would put all this insanity behind me. That was usually after watching an episode of NYPD Blue or Law and Order. I lived in a fantasy world concocted in my head and the idea of me being a cop at that stage of my life was farfetched at best. It sounded great and looked great on paper, but it wouldn't be long before reality would set in. As awesome as she was to be with, I couldn't be around her sober. I couldn't do anything sober at that point and it was becoming increasingly harder to function at all without alcohol and some form of opiate in my system. One Saturday night we went out in Bay Ridge with Patty and the girl he was seeing at the time. I went outside to pee because I was terrified of crowded bathrooms. I wound up nodding out standing up against a wall in the alleyway of a building around the block from the bar. By the time I came too it was an hour and a half later. I walked back into the bar like nothing happened. That was the first time she gave me that all too familiar look that people had been giving me for the last few years. I knew that look and I quickly went into survival mode. As fucked up as I was, I still had a way with words and could talk my way out of a lot of situations. I couldn't tell you what I said. I can only say that it worked. We wound up having a great night. Later on that night after we got home, we were sitting on my porch smoking a cigarette and she told me she loved me. I said the same and all was right with the world.

It was our "one month" anniversary we defiantly said to each other *"they said we wouldn't last four days, now it's four weeks, we showed them."* I used a gift card that someone gave me for my birthday to buy her a watch from Macys. It wasn't much but It was all I could do. I wasn't about to use the money I stole for drugs to buy her a gift so this seemed like the next best thing. We were changing it up this weekend. Her parents were going away so I was going to Long Island. I would take the train and she would pick me up after work and we'd spend the weekend at her house. It was great timing because everybody in Brooklyn was up my ass about my drinking and drugging and running away seemed like a logical thing to do. I wanted to leave forever but two or three days should cool everybody down enough for me to bullshit them to death when I got back. I had to make sure I was prepared so I stocked up on Oxy and Valium. I took what I thought was enough for three days. I popped three 80's and bought four Bud tall boys for the train ride. I felt great by the time I got there. I was getting away from my mess in Brooklyn, getting to see the person I loved to be around the most, and I was high as a kite. She picked me up and I couldn't wait to give her the watch. When she opened it, her eyes lit up and she cried a little. I had been hurting people on a regular basis for such a long time that it made me feel good to make someone else feel good for a change. We went to her house, got changed, and went out to some place I can't remember the name of. It was a big arcade which I'm not really into, but it had a bar and if it had a bar it didn't really matter where I was. We drank, laughed, hugged, and kissed. It really was a great time. When we woke up the next day she asked what I wanted to do and I said get drunk and lay here all day. I think those words hit home with her. I got that look from her again, the one she gave me the night I left her in the bar, and she was quiet the rest of the afternoon.

I said earlier I took enough Oxy and Valium for three days. The problem is that when I start I don't stop. The three days-worth of pills were gone by Saturday evening. While she was upstairs taking a shower, I did what I do. I started going through cabinets in search of what I needed. I couldn't be there straight and the alcohol wasn't enough. I hit the jackpot. I found a bottle of her father's Vicodin in the kitchen cabinet. At first, I took five or ten, but then I said to myself, five or ten isn't enough so let me just take the whole bottle and I'll replace them with some generic extra strength Tylenol. He'll notice five or ten missing, but he'll never know the difference if the bottle is full. Even if he does it would be weeks or months from now before he realized, and I'd deal with it then. I wound up stealing sixty Vicodin. The good thing was that now I didn't have to drink as much. I told her I was sorry for what I said earlier, and I didn't need to be drunk to have a good time with her. I must have been believable because the rest of the weekend was a blast. Monday morning came and she drove me to the train station. I didn't want to leave her, and I didn't want to face what was waiting for me at home. The money, Valium and Oxy I took with me was all stolen from my mother and aunt. I knew they knew because there were thirty voicemails telling me "we had to talk" when I got back. It was back to reality and I wasn't looking forward to it at all. We said our goodbyes and I headed for the train. I stopped in the deli and got my tall boys. I popped whatever Vicodin I had left and settled in for the trip home. I got on that train knowing that no matter what I had to deal with when I got home it would be ok because I would see Gina in a few days. What I didn't know then is that weekend and that goodbye in the car would be the last goodbye and I would never see Gina in that way again.

I got home from Long Island late that night. Everyone was already asleep. Between the long train ride home, the pills and booze I had been taking all weekend I just wanted to get in my bed and pass out. When I woke up the next day there was a note from my mother telling me not to leave until she got home to talk to me. My Aunt was in Pennsylvania for a few more days so the house was empty. I was shaky and needed to get right. I still had a few bucks left over from the weekend so I went to the store and bought six tall boys. I went up to my aunt's apartment to look for some Oxy and all she had was some five milligram Percs. They were catching on to my game and the hiding spots were becoming more creative. The Oxycontin was usually locked up or physically on her person. I found these Percs in an empty McDonalds soda cup on her dresser. I guess she figured I wouldn't look there, but the truth was I looked everywhere until

I found what I needed. I took a few Percs and washed them down with the tall boys. By the time my mother came home I was perfectly right and ready for the riot act I was about to be read. It was more of the usual. She would tell me how disappointed she was. She would tell me I was hurting everyone around me. She would tell me I was just like my father and ask why I did the things I did. I usually had all the answers mostly consisting of the *poor me, my life didn't turn out the way I wanted, so therefore I am the way I am.* This time I had no answers. I just sat there, took all she had to give and walked away without saying a word. I knew everything she said was right. I knew all the things I was doing were wrong, but at that point I had no answers and to be perfectly honest I didn't care. I even asked her for money to go out to the bar. I thought she was going to kill me. I went upstairs, took the few Percs I had left and waited for her to go to her room. As soon as she did I went downstairs and grabbed a hundred dollars in twenties out of her bag. I got dressed and made my phone calls. An hour later I was at the bar with a gram of coke and fifty dollars to drink with. I can't imagine the hurt and pain I caused her, but in the moment, I was blind to it. I was completely indifferent to anyone around me and how my actions were affecting them.

I got home around 2 am and I got on the computer and started chatting with Gina. She asked why I didn't answer the phone when she called earlier. I told her I wasn't feeling well and fell asleep early. I knew she'd hear it in my voice if I called her back so this was the best way to communicate. When I asked her if she was coming Friday she said she wasn't sure because of work. The four weeks prior this girl would work a twelve hour shift then drive an hour and a half to Brooklyn every day. It seemed a little strange to me that work may keep her away this weekend, but I was fueled up on a lot of coke and corona, so I didn't think too much of it. We said our goodnights and I slid into my nightly routine. I took a shower, popped a few Valiums and drank beers while watching tv until I passed out.

That Friday I was looking forward to seeing Gina. It was all I had to look forward to at this point. The hours passed and there was no word from her. She wasn't answering her phone, so I went on the computer to see if she was signed on. To my surprise she was. I asked her if she was coming and she said no. I asked if she was coming the next day and she said she didn't know. I got a nervous feeling in the pit of my stomach. I saw where this was going. She had been acting weird all week and now she was getting short with her answers. I had to give it one more test. I ended the chat with an I love you and a wink. I got nothing back. When I pushed the issue she just said, *"I don't know"*. I said *"what don't you know? You wither love me or you don't."* By now we were on the phone and I was getting increasingly agitated and my words were becoming desperate. How could she do this to me? A week ago it was us against the world. We spent three days planning our future. What could have changed so much in a few short days? Did someone get in her head? Did her father find out about the Vicodin? So many thoughts ran through my head. The reality was what everyone had warned from day one. I was a drunk and a junkie and she was a young girl coming off a recently ended relationship. She got excited to be with her childhood crush and it helped her fill a hole left by the breakup. When she realized what I was and how I was living she did what any sensible person would do. She ended it.

I was reaching for anything that would give my life some purpose, to fill the hole I had been filling with booze and drugs for so long. It never stood a chance. Normally, if you mess around with someone for a month or two and it doesn't work out you move on. You may be a little upset for a few days, but you move on. It is part of life. You live and learn. Unfortunately for me and most in active addiction everything is magnified tenfold. I felt hurt and betrayed. I felt like someone ripped a piece of my soul out. My stomach turned my body felt flush with adrenaline and I needed to make the hurt go away. I remember vividly walking quietly up to my aunt's apartment. By now it was past midnight and she was out cold. I needed to get some Oxycontin and I knew she would have them somewhere close to her so I couldn't get at them. I can't imagine having to live like that, not being able to keep your stuff in a drawer or medicine cabinet like a normal person because you have someone in your house that steals from you every chance he gets. I have two nephews now that I love like they're my own children, much like the love my aunt felt for me. The thought of them doing something like that to me makes me cringe, yet there I was looking at one of the two women who raised me as nothing more than an obstacle in the way of me getting what I needed. I even resented her for making it harder than it had to be. People aren't normally present when I'm on these missions so I needed to quietly search for the pills. There I was at twenty-seven years old crawling like a toy soldier across her living room floor and into her bedroom, creeping just feet away from her. At any moment she could've opened her eyes and seen her nephew, her Godson, a man she helped raise, rifling through her things like a crazed maniac, trying desperately to get the fix he needed to deal with the hurt he couldn't process. She didn't wake up and I found what I needed. They were right on top of her purse. I took what I needed and quickly left. I don't even remember how many I took or how much I drank, but I wound up at Patty's sister Kelly's house a few blocks away. Kelly was always someone I could talk to. I remember being sixteen and seventeen years old sitting on her porch, smoking cigarettes, talking about my how much my father leaving was bothering me or my girl problems of the week. If Patty and Joey were like my brothers she was most certainly like my sister. Her and her husband Ralph never turned me away no matter how crazy things got. I remember sitting at her kitchen table with a giant mug of beer. It had to be six in the morning. Her kids were very young at the time and I was a mess, but she listened to me and she calmed me down. I was very unstable from the mix of oxy and alcohol in my system, so she let me lay on the couch for a few hours. I look back in these moments and wonder what these people must have been going through seeing me like this. I can't imagine how hard it must have been on them. When I was finally able to stabilize enough to walk home I gave Kelly a hug and I thanked her. I don't remember what she said to me, but I do remember it was said with tears in her eyes. Nights like this would become more frequent and my downward spiral would only gain momentum from that day forward.

CHAPTER 15

Are You Jewish?

It was early October 2002. My use of Oxycontin was increasing, and I was up to four hundred milligrams a day, give or take, depending on my ability to steal them from my aunt. Back in the late 90's and early 2000's it wasn't like it is today. Nobody knew what Oxycontin really was, at least nobody that it was being prescribed to. It was being peddled as a miracle drug with no potential for addiction. This couldn't be further from the truth, as Oxycontin was nothing more than synthetic heroin in a pill form. I was about to find out just how similar the two were. It was a Monday or Tuesday afternoon and I had just taken my last pill. My uncle and cousin were over for dinner and I couldn't get into my aunt's apartment to get more. I thought to myself it's no big deal, I'll just get them tomorrow when my aunt goes to the doctor. Everyone left and I finished out my night as usual, with a few more beers and a benzo to put me to sleep. A few hours later I woke up in a pool of sweat, freezing cold. I didn't know what was wrong with me. I ran to the bathroom and threw up everything I had eaten for dinner and then it started coming out the other end. I was sitting on the bowl with my head in a small garbage pail cramping and heaving up every ounce of food and fluid that was in my body. All of a sudden I felt like I was on fire, thirty seconds later I was freezing. I jumped in the shower and put the water on as hot as I could get and it made me feel a little better, but I was still spraying fecal matter and vomit in every direction. It finally let up and I was able to clean myself off and bleach the shit out of the tub, literally and figuratively. I was freezing so I put on a big thick sweat suit went into my room and curled up in my bed. The next three days were more of the same. I had violent body cramps and I couldn't stop moving my legs. I had the chills one minute and the sweats the next. I had diarrhea and was throwing up nothing but yellow bile. I lost ten pounds in three days and there was a point that I really thought I was going to die. By this point I had my mother and aunt waiting on me hand and foot. They, like me, thought I was sick, maybe the flu, more likely food poisoning of some sort. I even conned my aunt into giving me an Oxycontin. I made her feel guilty. I pushed the theory that it was her food that put me in this awful situation, and because I had been throwing up so much, all my muscles locked up and I was in terrible pain. She gave me the pill and twenty minutes after I took it, I felt fine. No more aches, no more chills, no more stomach cramps, the urge to move my legs stopped. I was hungry and asked her to make me food. Twenty minutes before I was accusing her of poisoning me, now I'm asking for dinner. I didn't put two and two together, but that was my first experience of being dope sick. A week later I ran out of pills again and woke up with all the same symptoms. That's when it clicked. It was at that point that I knew I had a physical dependence on these little green pills. It was at that point that my brain said *you will never let yourself feel like this again.* By any means necessary I would get what I needed to not be sick. In recovery you hear about imaginary lines. It's often hard to distinguish exactly when things got out of control. I had crossed a thousand lines over the last ten years, but up until now I was just doing it to fit in, to feel different, to not feel at all, to kill the hurt, anger and guilt that had built up over the years, I liked being high because I hated myself when I wasn't. Now it was a different ballgame, now I needed these pills just to function. I needed them to get out of bed, to walk the dog, to eat and to talk to people. I needed these pills just to be normal. It wasn't about getting high anymore. To my brain it was about survival. It was an instinct, just like breathing.

I hadn't worked since losing my job at the firm and my mother was understandably up my ass to get a job. I was pretty much unemployable and to be honest I had lost all motivation to do anything but get high, which was in and of itself a full-time job. In stepped my Aunt Grace. Aunt Grace was my father's sister and in many ways was just like him. She was loud, charming and was never afraid to tell you exactly what was on her mind. She worked for a local councilman and got me my first job with at a local catering hall when I was fifteen. Everybody loved Grace. She was always shopping on "The Avenue" and held court like the she was the mayor of Bay Ridge. Everyone knew her and she stopped and talked to them all. She never cooked, so her and my Uncle Tony would go out to eat every night. Their favorite place was the Tiffany Diner in Bay Ridge and when that closed it was the Vegas Diner in Bensonhurst. She made my poor uncle split his meal with her every night. She had very short hair and would wrap a kerchief around her head wherever she went. My father would make fun of her calling her Francesca and ask her why she was always wearing a babushka. She was always cold and always made the diner turn down the air conditioning. No matter how hot it was outside and how many other patrons complained, they always obliged. That was Grace and Grace loved me. I mean she really thought the sun shined out of my ass. She had two daughters and couldn't stand my half-brother from my father's first marriage, so I was her boy. She used to take me to lunch with her friends when I was young and brag about how smart and handsome I was. She knew I was down on my luck, but not the reasons why. She called me one day and gave me the number of a friend of hers who managed a bank in Borough Park and told me to call for an interview. I needed to do something, and as messed up as I was, I could still make a good first impression, so I agreed to give her friend a call.

The interview was on a Thursday morning so I stopped drinking early Wednesday night so I wouldn't smell like booze the next day. I made sure I had enough Oxy to get myself right. I ironed my favorite navy-blue pinstriped suit, and I was ready to go. The next day I woke up and chewed two 80's. I swallowed one and drank a hot cup of tea. I walked into that place full of caffeine and Oxy, turned on the charm, and twenty minutes was all it took to win the manager over. I convinced her that I left wall street because I didn't like the cutthroat style. I told her that I spent the last eight months living off my savings trying to figure out what I wanted to do with my life. The fact that I was recommended by my Aunt helped, and I was offered the job on the spot. I would start the following Monday. The base salary wasn't great, but there were plenty of incentives to boost my pay. I was excited and I had every intention of giving this a real shot. Maybe this is what I needed. Maybe a reason to get up in the morning would help me get my shit together. I wanted to start straight. I had four days to kick the Oxy. I knew if I stopped that day, I would more than likely be ok by Monday. I went home and told my mother and Aunt Eileen that I got the job. They were thrilled. They were looking for any glimmer of hope for me, and this was the first glimmer in a long time. I called my Aunt Grace and thanked her, and then I settled in for what I knew was going to be a rough few days. I was prepared this time. I copped twenty Xanax from my friend Ronny, bought Nyquil, Gatorade, and Imodium and basically put myself into a coma for three days, only getting up to go to the bathroom and hydrate myself. By Sunday morning I was over the physical part of it and the Xanax dulled the mental anxiety and depression that usually followed. I ate a good lunch and dinner, took a nice hot shower, shaved, and settled into bed around nine o'clock. I was ready to go. I was ready to succeed. I was going to show everyone that I wasn't the useless, conniving junkie they all thought I was. Tomorrow would be a new beginning.

The bank was only twenty blocks away from my house. I could either take the train for a few stops or just walk. I felt better than I thought I would after kicking Oxy all weekend and the weather was decent, so I decided to walk and soak in some fresh morning air before I started my new life. I got there a half hour early and met a few of my co-workers. There was Kerry, a pretty black girl from Flatbush who aspired to run the place one day, Alex, a tiny little Puerto Rican girl from Sunset Park, Olga, a brutish Russian lady who lived in the neighborhood and then there was Yuri. Yuri was a thirty-year-old Russian Jew from Bensonhurst. He was the loudest dude I ever met in my life. When he said my name he screamed it. When he said anything, he screamed it. I found out later in the day that he was partially deaf in one ear. That explained the ungodly decibel levels his voice was at all the time. I liked Yuri from the minute I met him and we became fast friends. Concetta walked in around twenty minutes after I got there. Concetta or Connie was the manager I interviewed with the week before. She was a stout little Italian lady with fiery reddish hair. She looked the part of a bank manager. She was very personable and always dressed impeccably. As far as bosses go, she was a good one.

It was day one and we were about to have our morning meeting. I remember these being done at my old firm, but I was always so out of it I never paid any attention. I was turning over a new leaf today, so I was as attentive as I ever was for the twenty-minute rundown of the days plan. I would be training with Kerry the first day. She was the head customer service rep. In a bank you pretty much have tellers and customer service people. Customer service is where you want to be. The base salary was about the same, but with customer service came a desk, a phone, and a better opportunity to make some extra money selling bank products and insurance packages. I was still an egomaniac with the self-esteem of a flea so calling myself a bank teller is not something I wanted to do. Customer service liaison sounded a lot better. Long story short Connie told me I would be sitting with Kerry that day and then I would be training as a teller for the rest of the week so I could start on my own the week after. I'm a smart guy. I graduated Pace University with 2.5 GPA. I had a Major in Business Management and minors in Business Law, Finance and Accounting. I did this while being drunk every day for five years and physically going to a total of a maybe a hundred classes. I estimate that as around twenty percent effort. Fifty percent and I'm graduating with fifty Greek words next to my name. I was very confident that I could do enough in a week to prove I was worthy of a customer service desk.

The day started and the customers started rolling in. I mentioned that the bank was in Borough Park. Borough Park is almost exclusively inhabited by Hasidic Jews. They are deeply religious, deeply loyal to their families and community, very politically powerful and keenly aware of every penny that goes in and out of every transaction they make. Dealing with them can be difficult, especially if you are an outsider to their community. The first customer of the day was a man who wanted to open a congregation account. A Congregation account is basically a church account. It is a way for them to take in donations without being taxed. There were fifty of them being opened every day. I thought it was odd, but I didn't know enough to question it. Anyway, Kerry was giving the guy a hard time because he didn't have the right documentation. You needed IRS papers and a business ID to open one of these accounts and this guy didn't have either one. Connie didn't like to be involved with customers unless it was absolutely necessary. I could see Kerry was starting to lose her cool. The man was getting increasingly loud and Connie was starting to notice. Kerry had enough and she got up to seek Connie's assistance. There I was on my first day, not knowing the difference between a congregation account and a can of coke, left with this irate Jewish man, a pen and my notepad.

And vat do you think about this? he asked, in his heavy Jewish accent.

Sir, I have no idea, it's my first day. I replied.

First day, huh, Are you Jewish? He asked.

No sir, I'm Italian. I replied.

Vell, you look Jewish, it must be the nose. He replied, as he let out a huge belly laugh.

Vats your name? he asked.

Tommy. I replied.

Vell Tommy, I'm Moishe. It's nice to meet you. Do you smoke? I need a cigarette.

Yes, I do Moishe, let's go.

I went outside with Moishe to smoke a cigarette. Connie and Kerry were looking at us with dumbfounded confusion written all over their faces. Twenty minutes later I walked into the bank and sat down at Kerry's desk not saying a word. Connie walked over and they were both staring at me intently, waiting to hear what I had to say. I looked up at both of them like nothing had just happened and said,

Is there something I can help you with?

What happened out there? Kerry asked.

Yes, what happened? Connie asked, still looking confused.

Oh, you mean with Moishe? I asked sarcastically.

YESSSSSSSSSS. Both ladies shouted.

He'll be back tomorrow with all his paperwork. I replied very nonchalantly.

What did you say to him? Connie asked.

Nothing. I replied.

We just had a cigarette.

Both ladies laughed with relief. They could not believe it. Yuri screamed my name right in my ear as he pounded his hand on my back. Apparently, Moishe was the biggest pain in the ass customer in the neighborhood. He had twenty-five accounts at the bank and never had the correct paperwork to open any of them. He thought because he had a lot of money in the bank, he could do whatever he wanted. The truth is we just bullshitted about baseball and the stock market. I told him to come back tomorrow with the right paperwork and I would personally take care of him. I apologized for the inconvenience and explained to him that we had a meeting that morning and were told that the IRS was cracking down on congregation accounts and we really had to cross our t's and dot our i's going forward. It was a complete crock of shit. I finally used my conniving ways for good and it worked. Connie told me I would be training with Kerry the rest of the week and get my own desk the following Monday. Less than an hour in the place and I already won them all over. Any time I put the effort in I succeeded in life, especially when I wasn't stoned out of my mind. I felt good about myself for the first time in a long time. I felt so good I bought a six pack of tall boys on the way home. I said to myself, *I deserve it, I was a fucking superstar today.* I went home and laid on my couch sipping on the frosty cold Budweiser. I was so tired that I only drank three. That may have been the first time in ten years I didn't finish all the beer I bought. I took shower and laid in my bed. As I was falling asleep, I thought to myself, *this is what it's all about. I worked hard today, and I did good. I came home and drank like a normal person. If I can just do this everything will be ok.* As I faded off to sleep, I really thought it was going to be all good from that day on.

CHAPTER 16

A Junkie and a Russian Walk into a Bar

Things were going great at the bank. I was on my own midway through the first week. Yuri had a family commitment, so they needed me to take some customers on my own. It was my moment to shine and that's exactly what I did. I opened six accounts by lunch and had the customers eating out of my hand. At the end of my first week Connie called me into her office and told me how surprised she was that I caught on so quickly. She was impressed and happy to have me as part of her team. That made me feel good. Less than a year before, I had disappointed everyone at the firm. I disappointed my family, my friends and was very close to facing serious legal consequences. I had all the ingredients to be a star, but I let alcohol and drugs wash all the promise away. Now ten months later my potential was shining through. I spoke earlier about telling Patty on the way home from a trip to hunter mountain, that all I needed was a good job and a nice girl to turn my life around. I finally had the first of the two. It was the Friday night of my first week at the bank and everyone was hanging out at G's. I grabbed a twelve pack of Corona and headed there after work. I drank and smoked weed until three in the morning, then went home to bed. Saturday I did the same. Sunday was softball in the morning and over to Joey and Patty's for football and beers the rest of the day. It was a good weekend. I didn't get crazy. I didn't do any hard drugs and I went to sleep at a normal hour on Sunday. I was getting the hang of this normal life thing and I was happy.

I continued to excel at work. The customers were getting to know me and some of them were asking to see only me. The Hasidic community is very interesting to say the least. Every day people would come in and cash eighteen dollar checks by the dozens. If it wasn't eighteen it would be a multiple of eighteen. One day I asked one of them what the deal was with the eighteen dollars. He told me it was a good luck thing. In Hebrew, letters have numerical values. The number 10 is the letter Yud. The number 8 is the letter Het. Het-Yud spells the word Chai which means life. When someone gives eighteen dollars or a multiple of, it symbolizes giving life or luck to the recipient. I found that fascinating. When I asked Kerry the day before, she told me it was because they were cheap. That's why I was good at my job. I took the time to learn about my customers. I learned that from John when I worked at Foleys. He told me to know what all my regulars drink and have it ready for them before they ask. Learn about their lives and their families. When you show interest in people, they feel comfortable with you. In turn, they will take an interest in you. I had one couple that owned a vitamin store. Whenever they had a new product they would bring me a bottle to try. The man across the street knew I liked tuna. I would go into his store three times a week at lunchtime and order tuna on a bagel with pickles. If I was busy and didn't get there by a certain time, he would call me and ask if I was hungry. If I said yes, he would bring the sandwich over and tell me that a young man must eat. I really enjoyed working there and it showed. My family was thrilled with my behavior. I would bring my aunt and mother flowers on Fridays. For the first time in a long time I would give my mother money to help with the house. They put up with a lot and they deserved some peace in their lives. Life was good.

I had been at the bank for about six weeks. Me and Yuri stayed late one Thursday night to call some customers and pitch our insurance products. That night we were on fire. Each of us scheduled three appointments for the following week and I even got one lady to purchase a long-term care policy over the phone. We finished up around eight o'clock and Yuri suggested we go out for a few drinks. I hadn't been out to a bar in a while and Yuri was fun to hang out with so I said yes and we headed to Bay Ridge. The name of the bar was either Raspberries or Cranberries and it was attached to a dive hotel. The hotel was not a five-star spot. It was one with hourly rates, frequented by addicts, prostitutes and people with nowhere else to go, that lived there for days or months at a time. The bar was no better. It was esthetically nice inside, but the place was seedy. I had been in enough bars over the years to know the type of place this was. Yuri knew the owner and had done some promotions for the place, so I gave it a shot. Being around that environment brought about certain feelings. I had been towing the line for a month and a half now, drinking very moderately and smoking weed here and there. Being in this place triggered some urges. Three screwdrivers and two coronas in twenty minutes didn't help the situation. Yuri knew me from work. He knew the good me. He saw that I was a little anxious and told me to loosen up and have some fun. This poor guy had no idea who he was talking to. We started talking to these two girls. When they asked what we did I jumped in before Yuri could speak and said that we were financial advisors. Their eyes lit up and they were ready to party. The bells were going off in my head and I wanted some coke. I had an uncanny ability to find drugs. Brinsley used to say that I could be in a room of ten thousand saints and I would find the one degenerate with drugs and he was right. Twenty minutes and three conversations later I had two eight balls and eight hits of ecstasy. Yuri looked at me like I was crazy, and I said,

"You told me to loosen up pal. Everything from here on out is your fault. Now get ready to have some fucking fun."

The girls lived in the neighborhood and asked us to come back and party with them. Me and Yuri went to the store to get some beer and met them at their apartment. It was a nice place on the first floor of a two-family house. The girls turned out to be strippers. I used to hang out with two strippers that lived a few blocks away from me. I hung out with them strictly because they got great cocaine for free and had a big monster of a bodyguard named Bo that would drive me all over the place when they were working. I felt like a gangster walking into bars with this guy. He was awesome, but those girls were dirtbags. Their apartment was infested with roaches and the whole building smelled like garbage. The girls tonight weren't dirtbags. The place was clean, and they were nice girls. We started playing some drinking games and doing lines of cocaine. At this point, Yuri realized he was in a little over his head. He was wrecked and kept asking me when we were leaving. I still had a few grams of coke left and eight hits of ecstasy, plus we were off the next day because we had both worked the previous Sunday. In Borough Park, banks are closed on Saturday and open on Sunday. If you worked on a Sunday you would get a day off during the week. I wasn't close to done. I told him to do a few lines to sober up. He was hesitant at first, but he eventually gave in. Yuri was loud to begin with, now he was like a megaphone. We were having a blast.

The girls were getting increasingly flirtatious and I saw this night heading in a very good direction. That's when it happened. I noticed an orange pharmacy bottle in one of the girl's bags. I got up to get a beer and noticed they were forty milligram Oxycontin. I hadn't had an OC in a while. As soon as I saw them my stomach got tight and I became excited like a little kid coming down to a living room full of presents on Christmas morning. I was going to ask for one, but I didn't want one, I wanted them all. They wanted to take the ecstasy, so I gave them two hits each and pretended to take one myself. I told Yuri we weren't going to take any because I had a plan. I told him to be ready when I said it was time to go. About an hour later these girls were rolling their faces off. Anyone who has taken ecstasy knows it's a very sexual drug and these two were ready to go. They were practically begging us to have sex with them. Here I am with two beautiful girls ready to do whatever I wanted. We had a bunch of alcohol, ecstasy and coke and all I can think about is the bottle of pills in the girl's bag. Yuri was making out with one of the girls on the couch. The other girl was feeling nauseous from the ecstasy and when she got up to go to the bathroom I saw my opportunity. As soon as she left the room I grabbed the bottle of Oxy and put it in my pocket. I tapped Yuri's girl on the leg and told her to go check on her friend. As soon as she turned the corner of the hallway I grabbed Yuri and said,

> *"Let's get the fuck out of here bro."*
> *"What do you mean get the fuck out of here, we're about to get laid."* He screamed as only Yuri could.
> *"Fuck getting laid man, we gotta go."* I said as I pulled him toward the door.

By now the girls heard Yuri's big mouth and asked what was going on.

> *"Yuri, please bro, I will explain everything in the car, I promise you, but right now we have to go."*
> *"Okay, okay man, but you owe me a girl."* He replied.

I couldn't help but laugh. He was like a kid who just lost his puppy. I felt bad for him. He was so close and I snatched it right from under him. We finally got out of the apartment and ran down the block towards his car. All I heard were the two girls yelling out the window asking where we were going. We left all the coke and ecstasy, but I didn't care. I hit the mother load. It was a newly filled bottle of forty milligram OC's. There were sixty of them. As Yuri dropped me off on the corner of my block, he looked at me and said,

"Bro, what the fuck was that all about?" You better have some good reason for pulling the shit you just pulled."

"Right here my friend, these pills are worth a fortune on the street." I replied.

I was full of shit. I wasn't about to sell a single one of those pills. I had been off them for a while now so sixty pills would last me two months. At least that's what my sick mind was telling me in that moment. Yuri looked at me with disgust, I was ready for him to call me a junkie dirtbag and kick me out of his car. He would tell everyone at work what happened and the job I loved so much would be gone. Just as quickly as I earned the reputation as a solid guy and a great worker is just as quickly it would disappear. I would be looked at as a lowlife. I would disappoint everyone again and be back to square one. Only that's not what happened. Yuri looked at me with disgust and said,

"That's why you dragged me out of there you mother fucker. I can get you those things cheap anytime you want. My cousin Ilya works at a pharmacy, he can get whatever you want."

My eyes popped like a deer in headlights, I wanted to hug him. I apologized to him and promised him next time we went out I would find him the hottest girl in the place and pay for the whole night. He looked at me and said,

"Yea, Yea. Get out of my car you motherfucker, we'll talk Monday."

I got out of the car and walked up to my house. I did a lot of coke that night and the adrenaline from stealing the pills and racing out of the place had me amped up. There was no way I was falling asleep on my own. I found a Xanax in my drawer and took it. I washed it down with one of the tall boys that I still had in my fridge from that first night I worked at the bank. Six weeks of being good, six weeks of being happy and six weeks of showing everyone I could be a productive human being were out the window. I realized as I was laying in my bed staring at the ceiling that I was right back to where I started. One night is all it took. I could go in the bathroom right now and flush the OC's, or even better go back to the girl I stole it from and give it back. She could've really needed them. I could stop this before it started. One night isn't so bad. Sure, I went a little crazy, but Yuri wasn't going to tell anyone. I've never seen those two girls before and I'll probably never see them again. I could stop now and start over again tomorrow. I could wake up Monday and go back to work and continue to move forward with my life. That all sounded nice in my head, but I didn't do any of it. The monster was awake and the only thing I could do was get up the next day and feed it what it wanted.

I could tell you that I was proud of myself for not taking any of the Oxy I stole from the girls the next day, but that was because I slept through the next day. Thankfully, my mother and aunt were in Pennsylvania. I didn't have to explain why I slept for twenty hours straight, only getting up to pee. The only time I did that was when I was detoxing. This was just from exhaustion and an absurd amount of alcohol and coke the night before. The first thing I did when I woke up was pop an Oxy. Having not taken any since early October, one pill would get me where I wanted to go. I drank some coffee and went down to Joe's deli for a toasted bagel and a six pack of tall boys. I spent Saturday on my couch doped up on Oxy, drinking beer and watching reruns of NYPD Blue. I kept my promise to myself of only taking two pills. I took one more at around five o'clock. I went to Patty's house to drink some more beer and we wound up at the Wicked Monk later that night. It was a fun and mellow night. I got home around three in the morning and went right to sleep.

Softball was over, so I figured why not start off my day with two pills. Even if I took one more later that day it would still be far less than I was taking before I started working at the bank. I wound up taking five that Sunday. Two hundred milligrams was still less than what I was previously on, but in two short days I was on the fast track to the same situation I was in six weeks earlier. The thing about Oxy is, if you didn't go overboard and stayed within a limit, you can be very productive. I've had some of my most physically productive moments in life while on Oxy. I got up Monday morning and I was already feeling a slight withdrawal. I chewed one for the quick rush and swallowed the other for the sustained high throughout the day. I put two more in my pocket just in case and by ten o'clock I was in the bathroom crushing one up on the toilet paper dispenser. Three days and I'm already out of control. I'm chewing them, I'm sniffing them at work, but I'm still telling myself that I'm being productive. It hasn't taken hold of me yet and because of that I told myself I would be fine. I told myself it made me better at my job and at life.

Yuri was on the mid-day shift. I was in the break room eating lunch when he came into the room like he was shot out of a cannon.

Tommy, we have to talk bro." He bellowed in Yuri volume.
"What's up Pal?"

I answered very calmly, as calm as a guy who just sniffed another forty milligrams of Oxy. I was feeling no pain. It was noon and I had only been up for five hours, but I was already a hundred and sixty milligrams deep. This is where you aren't productive. This is where you nod out on the break room couch and throw up in the bathroom for the last twenty minutes of your lunch break.

"Come on guy, snap out of it. If Connie sees you like this she'll lose her shit." He said.

"I'm fine bro, my back hurt this morning so I took one of those pills." I replied.

I convinced him that because I hadn't taken any in so long that my tolerance was low. That was partially the truth. I asked him to grab me a cup of coffee so I could wake myself up a little before I went back upstairs. He obliged, and we talked about the Thursday night adventure we had.

"Tommy, you're a sick bastard. What kind of guy robs two girls before he gets laid?" He asked.

This guy was still mad that I made him run out of there before he got some.

"Yuri, for the tenth time, I'm sorry, I will make it up to you. It was too good an opportunity and it had to be done that way."

He finally looked like he accepted my apology. He told me he spoke to his cousin and he wanted to meet me and discuss some business. I completely forgot about his cousin. Bells started going off in my head. When I'm using there is never enough. If I have a million pills, I will start wondering what I'm going to do when I run out after I take the first one. I had sixty on Saturday and I was already down to fifty by lunchtime on Monday. Yuri's cousin wanting to talk to me was music to my ears. It was a week before Christmas, and we decided to go to the Staten Island Mall the next day and do some shopping. Yuri's cousin would meet us there.

The following night we went to the mall straight from work. Yuri bought a watch for a girl he was seeing. I had nobody to buy for. Gina had dumped me a couple of months earlier and I hadn't started seeing anyone new. I had already gotten gifts for my mom, aunt and cousin. The only other people I got gifts for were Kelly's three kids and they were always gift cards. The only reason I was there was to meet Ilya. An hour after we got there he showed up. Ilya seemed to be the opposite of Yuri. He was a little conservative looking guy. He dressed very professional and wore a Yamaka on his head. He was very soft spoken and polite, at least I thought he was. The first thing I said to him was that there was no way they were related. He got a laugh out of that and we started our conversation.

"My cousin tells me you wanted to talk." He said.
"I absolutely do." I replied.
"Yuri tells me that you have a connection in the Pharmacy business." I continued.
"I don't have a connection." He replied.

My heart dropped. Yuri wasted my time. My mind immediately went into panic mode. I started thinking of the impending detox from the Oxy. I was already at a two hundred milligram a day pace and it was progressing every day. I thought to myself, this is his revenge for Thursday. This mother fucker got my hopes up just to watch them come crashing down. After about a minute of uncomfortable silence Ilya chimed in.

"I am the connection mother fucker, let's talk business."

That's when I realized that Ilya was just like Yuri. He wasn't loud and obnoxious, but he had a very sarcastic wit about him. Like Yuri, I liked Ilya almost immediately.

I started off asking what he could get, how often, what quantities and how much it cost. He looked at me with a straight face and said,

"Whatever you need I can get. However many you want I can get. Whenever you need them, I will have them for you."

Part of me was expecting a cameraman to pop out of nowhere and tell me I was on some practical joke show. I figured I'd start small and test the waters on my first order. I asked him for fifty Valium and fifty OC 80's. He told me the 80's were hard to get, but he could definitely get the 40's. I agreed and asked what the price was going to be. He told me it would be seven hundred for everything. I did some quick math. Fifty OC 40's had about a two-thousand-dollar street value. Fifty Valium had between a fifty and a hundred-dollar street value depending on the strength. I knew I was making out like a bandit, but I had to question the thought process behind the figure.

"Where did you come up with that number?" I asked.

"Seven dollars a pill is the price, I'm taking a big risk here. You don't like the price you can go somewhere else, or better yet you can keep robbing strippers." He fired back aggressively.

"Take it easy Scarface." I replied jokingly.

I realized that he had no idea what the OC's were worth, so I just let him think he was getting over on me.

"Seven hundred it is."

I glared over in Yuri's direction. He looked like he wanted to crawl into a garbage can. Ilya was most certainly not supposed to bring the stripper thing up to me. I swore Yuri to secrecy about that whole situation. Yuri knew I was pissed. How am I supposed to trust this guy? We go out one night, commit one crime and he can't wait to spill the beans to the first person who would listen. I told Ilya to meet me by the bank the next day with the pills and I would have the money. As he was leaving, he had one more request. He wanted me to take the hold off some checks that he received from relatives that lived out of the country. He got these checks every week and because they were foreign there was a seven day hold on the funds. Why he was getting these checks I have no idea. I asked why his cousin couldn't do it. He said it would look suspicious if Yuri was the only person dealing with him in the bank. I agreed to do it. We shook hands and started to go our separate ways. Just as he turned to walk away, I called out to him.

> *"Ilya, when you come into the bank tomorrow come straight to my desk. If I'm with someone just wait for me. Put the pills in an envelope or a paper bag. Give me the checks and I'll bring them up to the teller and sign off on the hold removal. When I'm up there, drop the pills in the slot on my desk that goes to the garbage can. When I come back, I will put your cash and receipts in an envelope that I will grab from my top drawer. Your five hundred will be in there."*

Ilya and Yuri both had confused looks on their faces. *"It's seven hundred Tommy."* Ilya said with a little bass in his voice.

> *"No Ilya, it's five. Two hundred is the price for bank fraud. If you don't like it, go to Western union and cash your checks. I'll see you tomorrow."*

I turned around and walked away. When we got in the car Yuri looked at me and just shook his head and smiled.

> *"You're really a sick bastard. I've never seen anyone get over on Ilya like that."* He said.

I looked over at him and in the calmest voice possible said.

"If you ever tell another person about what happened the other night, the next time your cousin sees you will be at your funeral. Are we clear with that?"

"We're good Tommy. My bad." He replied.

I settled back in the seat, popped another pill, closed my eyes and said,

"Good, now let's get the fuck out of here. I hate Staten Island."

CHAPTER 17

Ain't Nothing But a "G" Thing

I woke up the morning after the meeting with Ilya, excited. He set some big expectations and I was anxious to see if he could come through. I got dressed, sniffed two OC's, swallowed one and headed to the bank. I drank a huge cup of coffee when I got there and I was feeling lovely. I had the perfect amount of dope and caffeine coursing through my body. I opened ten accounts myself and helped Kerry with two of her own. If I could get the steady flow of Oxy that Ilya promised I would be unstoppable. I was in a full-blown euphoric fantasy land and I had no desire to come back to reality.

It was around eleven-thirty. I was eating lunch in the break room when Yuri came in to tell me his cousin was there to see me. I quickly finished my lunch and made my way upstairs, stopping briefly to go in the bathroom and sniff two more pills. Ilya played his part perfectly. He sat at my desk and handed me five checks totaling one thousand dollars. I filled out the deposit and withdraw slip and headed up to the teller. I went to Alex's station. I told her to deposit the checks into his account and withdraw one thousand in cash. As she was counting the money, I quickly removed the hold on her computer. She handed me the cash along with Ilya's receipt and I started walking back to my desk. As I counted out the cash to put into the envelope, I noticed something strange. The money Alex gave me seemed to be too much. I counted it twice. I couldn't believe what I was seeing. For whatever reason, Alex gave me two thousand dollars. My brain processed a hundred thoughts in the thirty seconds it took me to palm the extra thousand into my top drawer as I grabbed Ilya's envelope. Was I being set up? Was this a test they put all their employees through? Should I tell Alex? Should I tell Connie? What will happen if I take it and get caught? My mother would be ashamed. I would tarnish the reputation of my Aunt Grace, one more relative who made the tragic mistake of using their name to vouch for me. I would absolutely get locked up. Thought after thought led to the only conclusion my addict mind had the capability of coming to in that moment. I kept the money. I put Ilya's thousand in the envelope along with the five already in there for the pills. He took it. He shook my hand and smiled, motioning his eyes to the garbage slot on my desk and then left the bank. The transaction went off without a hitch. I quickly pretended to tie my shoe and removed the envelope, leaving it on the floor next to the pail. I didn't leave my desk the rest of the day. Between the drugs on the floor and the money in my drawer I was an anxious wreck. Yuri asked me if I was ok at least five times. I had a few more customers to take care of and thankfully none of them required me to do much work. Three o'clock came and we locked the doors.

The end of the day consisted of auditing our paperwork for all accounts we opened and the tellers reconciling their drawers. Connie spends that whole time with the tellers, making sure every penny is accounted for. This gave me the opportunity to get the envelope with the pills and put the thousand dollars of ill-gotten bank money in the garbage can. You may be asking yourself; *Why the fuck would he put a thousand dollars in the garbage?* Connie and Alex were going to find the discrepancy in Alex's receipts for the day. They were going to investigate. They were going to go through every transaction made that day. We would all come into question and the money would have to be answered for. By putting it in the garbage can I gave myself wiggle room. If things started pointing at me, I could easily throw the bag in the main pail. If they were desperate enough to go through the garbage, it would be found and chalked up to a careless mistake. If they decided it was foul play involving one of us, the proof was gone. I knew where every camera was in that place and where they were pointed. I wasn't on any of them when I palmed the cash or when I put it in my pail. I was completely insulated from any blame, unless of course it was a setup, in which case I was fucked anyway. At least I had my pills. In the end it was chalked up to teller error on a five-thousand-dollar withdrawal earlier in the day. Whatever method of deduction they used was obviously wrong and Alex wound up taking the hit. It wasn't life changing. The banks money is insured and she was given a verbal warning. I felt bad in the moment. Alex was a sweet girl and I found her crying in the break room when all was said and done. I told her it was no big deal and that everyone makes mistakes. I even went to the deli across the street and bought her a cup of the tea she drank every day. She hugged me and cried some more on my shoulder and thanked me for being so nice. By now the money was safely stashed in my sock and my pills were locked in my desk drawer. Part of me wanted to come clean. Part of me wanted to go with my original escape plan and throw the cash in the garbage, hoping for someone to look and find it and Alex would be off the hook. Those parts of me were long overtaken by the part that took the money in the first place.

I spent the next half hour talking Alex off the ledge, eventually joined by Yuri. Between the both of us, we had her laughing by the time we were ready to leave. Connie came down and read us the riot act, telling us to be more diligent in our work habits. When it was time to leave, Alex hugged me again and thanked me. Yuri slapped me on the back like only Yuri could and told me I was a good guy for talking to Alex the way I did. I went to my drawer and grabbed the pills I had yet to check for quality and quantity. As we left the bank and said our goodbyes, I thought to myself;

"You have them all fooled. They just thanked you for robbing them. There is nothing you can't pull off. You are a fucking Rockstar."

I didn't want to think that way, but that's who I was. When I first started that job, my mother said to watch my sticky fingers. She knew the temptation that exists working in a bank and having access to large sums of cash. That temptation exists for a normal person. She knew I was high risk and I kept that thought in my head. Up to that point the thought never crossed my mind, but on that day, when the opportunity found me, I took it without a second thought. It was easy and that was the worst part of it. It was too easy. Later that night I got home and checked my stash. It was fifty OC 40's and fifty ten milligram Valiums. The little bastard came through. Not only that, but I was also a thousand dollars richer. I immediately called Ilya and ordered a hundred more OC's. I was so hyped I called the two Joeys, G, Mikey and Patty and told them to meet me at Bennett's. I swallowed two OC's, sniffed two, and headed out. I was flush with cash, flush with drugs, and the feeling of invincibility was growing stronger by the minute.

Ilya's visits to the bank started becoming a regular thing. I was selling the bare minimum of the OC's just to be able to pay for my next reup. My reups were becoming so frequent that I started picking them up at his apartment to avoid suspicion. Half the time he wouldn't be home and his wife would count out the pills for me. I felt bad when his son would come out when the pills were being counted. A little kid shouldn't see stuff like that, but that didn't stop me. I was putting a lot of money in his pocket and he was keeping the beast in me fed. It was a mutually beneficial relationship, and I didn't want to mess that up by telling him his kid should stay in his room when we're doing our business. Problem is that I started using so much and selling so little that I was having a hard time coming up with the money to pay. I had to figure out a way to get money and what better place to do that than a bank.

It was mid-January. By now I was up to a four hundred milligram a day habit on top of a half a case of beer. It was getting harder to get to work every day and when I was there I could barely keep my eyes open. I had to start adding cocaine back into the mix just so I could get through the day. It was my turn to work the Sunday shift, and when I walked in, Alex was already there and in a full blown panic. She was supposed to order the money needed for Sunday before we left on Friday afternoon and she forgot. When Sunday came, we had no money in the bank. We reached out to the on-call manager and explained the situation. He told me that our other branch in the area would be able to give us enough to get through the day. He would pick me up in a half hour so we could go pick it up. This gave me time to go downstairs and sniff an OC and a few lines of coke. By the time he got there I was ready to run through a brick wall. We walked in the other branch and the girl behind the teller windows came out and handed me a satchel. Inside was one hundred and thirty-eight thousand dollars. I was in shock that they just transported this much money without any sort of security and the fact that they gave it to me was astonishing in my own head. If they only knew. I wanted to call one of my friends and tell them to come hit me in the head with a hammer and take the money. When I eventually woke up we would split the money. I played the whole thing out in my head and realized the chances of getting away with that were slim. I guess I got lost in my thoughts because the manager had pulled up in front of my branch and had to snap me back to reality with a shout of my name. I apologized and started to make my way out of the car. As I was exiting, my curiosity got the best of me.

"Hey, don't you get nervous moving this much money around?" I asked.

"No, it's not my money and it's not my fault they're too cheap to hire a security guard on the weekends. If anyone wants it they can have it. All of it is insured anyway. Have a good day kid. Call me if you need anything else."

With that he drove away. By now Yuri was there and the two of us helped Alex set up her teller station and me and Yuri got ourselves ready for the day ahead.

The day was slow. If we had thirty customers it was a lot. That was surprising for a Sunday, but I was perfectly ok with it. I was in the bathroom half of the day ripping lines of coke and oxy anyway. My brain kept going back to the words of the manager. The money is insured. Nobody will be hurt if it gets taken. Those words echoed in my head that entire day. The wheels started spinning. The amount I was carrying that day was too much. The bank is insured, but if over a hundred thousand goes missing there will be a lot of heat. If there was a way to do it in smaller increments it could probably go unnoticed.

Earlier that week we had done an audit of all inactive accounts at our branch to determine if they were to be declared dormant. Dormant accounts are ones that have had no activity in a certain period of time. Banks are required by law to report these accounts to the state after reasonable efforts have been made to contact the account holder. If the owner can't be contacted, the money is transferred to the state for safekeeping. They then take over the funds and the record keeping. After the audit, we were given a list of accounts that were about to go dormant and asked to contact the account holders to give them their final notice. Just like that it all clicked. Bells went off in my head like a slot machine hitting the jackpot on a quiet Sunday afternoon. It took me less than ten minutes to formulate a plan in my head and I would put it to the test the next day. This would be a game changer. It was risky and wrong on every level, but if it worked I would have unlimited access to funds and never have to worry about running out of pills again.

CHAPTER 18

But You Don't Work Here Anymore

I woke up bright and early the next day. I was about to put my plan into motion. I was nervous, as well as excited. There was a set of rules I put together that would give me less of a chance of getting caught as well. They would also ease the feelings of stealing money from innocent, unsuspecting people. They were as follows.

1. The account had to have over twenty thousand dollars in it. I didn't want to steal from someone who couldn't afford it.
2. It had to be a passbook account. People who get statements are more likely to check their balances. Passbooks only got updated when the person made a transaction.
3. The person on the account couldn't be over 65. I didn't want to steal from the elderly.
4. No beneficiary accounts and no college funds. I didn't want a kid to lose his inheritance or education because I needed to get my fix.

Aside from number two the rest were a crock of shit. I was stealing form my own friends and family. I couldn't give a fuck less about complete strangers. It just made me feel better about myself to think I had some semblance of a moral code left.

I arrived at work an hour early. I wanted to go through the list and vet out the candidates for my plan. I found two. Both were people in their fifties. Both were passbook savings accounts with over twenty thousand dollars in it and the best part is they didn't live in the area anymore. For the plan to work, the bank needed to be crowded. The tellers had to be busy and I needed two customers to be sitting at my desk. The customers would then need to make a withdrawal. The plan was to fill out a withdrawal slip in the name of the dormant account holder for nine hundred dollars. Anything over one thousand needed a manager approval. I would bring it to the teller with the slip for the real customer I was taking care of. When the bank is crowded and the tellers are busy, they don't pay too much attention to what transactions we process. If asked, I would tell her or him that each customer at my desk is making a withdrawal. I would have the nine hundred slightly separated by one finger from the rest of the money. When I went back to the desk, I would go into my top drawer to grab an envelope for the customers and drop the nine hundred. I would close the desk, give my customers their money, and walk them out the front door. It was risky and I knew I was taking a huge chance, but I didn't care. I needed to support my habit by any means necessary.

Four hours went by and nothing. Everyone came in singles and the one couple didn't make any withdrawal. Finally, at about one o'clock I got what I needed. Three men came in and two of them were making withdrawals. Three was a little tricky, but I needed to make this work, so I was giving it a shot no matter what. The bank was packed and the tellers were busy. I had the slip already filled out from earlier in the day. I walked behind the counter and handed Allah the three slips. As packed as it was, wouldn't you know it, she questioned it right away. With a passbook account you need to have the book with you so the bank can document the transaction. That part honestly slipped my mind and I had to think quick. I thought back to that day almost twenty years earlier when my father questioned me about the bat incident. I thought about the thousand other lies I told over the last ten years and with little hesitation I said,

"Mr. ---- left his passbook at his home in Jersey. He needs this money to give the down payment for the flowers for his daughter's wedding. He will bring the book in next week when he comes back."

She bought it hook, line and sinker. In her heavy Russian accent she said,

"Ok, only for daughter. Make sure he brings back next veek or there vill be penalty."

Lying became easy. I became so good at it that I believed half the shit I was saying. I guess that's what made it so believable. I brought the money to my desk and dropped the nine hundred in my drawer. I handed the two men envelopes with their money and the other man got an envelope with a bank brochure and my card. The plan went off without a hitch. By the end of that week, I had done this five more times. In total it was just a little over five thousand dollars and I bought twenty-five hundred dollars' worth of Oxycontin. Ilya balked at first, but when I told him I'd take my business elsewhere he said he could do it. Being it was so much, he told me he would have to do it in separate orders. The good news was that he was able to get the 80's for the first time. Every week for the next five weeks he would bring me a sealed bottle of one hundred pills. For the next five weeks I swallowed, chewed, snorted and smoked upwards of eight hundred milligrams of Oxycontin every day. I used the rest of the ill-gotten money to drink and sniff coke all night. One night I was out in Bay Ridge. I was out of my mind. I was speed balling coke and oxy for weeks now and I was becoming strung out. I wound up running into a friend from the neighborhood. His name was Davey. He was a good guy, but like me, he had his own issues with substance use. We wound up at an after hours in Borough Park where we met two girls. We decided we would go to the infamous Harbor Motor Inn on Shore Parkway to continue the party. The Harbor was your classic drug spot, and like the hotel I spoke about in Bay Ridge, it was inhabited largely by people doing exactly what we were there to do. We had so much booze and drugs that the girls were an afterthought. I couldn't care less if they were there or not. After an hour in the room of more vodka, cocaine and oxy, there was a knock at the door. The paranoia was insane and all of us except one girl were terrified of what was on the other side of that door. It turned out to be her boyfriend. I had seen him at the after hours earlier that night. This guy had a bad look about him and me and him didn't see eye to eye from the minute he walked in. After a half hour of him shooting deadly looks at me from across the room. I got up and said to him.

> *"Listen bro, I don't know what the fuck your problem is, but I want nothing to do with your girlfriend, I'm just here to get high. You can take those dirty looks and fuck off."*

You can't really blame the guy. His girlfriend was getting high with two dudes in a sleazy hotel. I normally wasn't like that, but it was the tail end of a week's long binge and I had no patience. With that he reached into his waste, pulled out what looked like a .38 revolver and pointed it six inches from my head. I wasn't expecting that. I should've been terrified, but I wasn't. All the noise in my head went away. I wouldn't have to do this anymore. No more lying, no more stealing, no more letting everyone I ever cared about down. In that moment I felt at peace. I closed my eyes, leaned my forehead into the gun and softly said,

> *"Pull the trigger bro, you'd be doing me a favor."*

At that moment Davey jumped up and started pleading with this guy to put his gun away. I couldn't tell you what he said, but it worked. The guy lowered the gun, grabbed his girl and left the room. I think my absolute willingness to die that night shook him. It shook me as well. I should've felt relieved, but I didn't. I felt like my out was right there and now I would have to keep on living this shit life I created for myself. I drank some more vodka, took some more Oxy and sniffed some more coke. I called my friend Jim to come pick me up. He had a hockey game that morning and said he would get me, but I had to come to the game. I sat there that Sunday morning, on the bench of a rink I once played on, strung out and upset that I didn't die the night before. Where did my life go? The worst part of a long drug fueled run is the end. When you run out of resources you are left with yourself. The depression is debilitating. All I could do that morning is finish the small amount of cocaine I had left and contemplate my next move. I needed more drugs, and I needed more money. I got home at noon, took a shower and passed out in my bed. I woke up nine hours later and I felt awful, but I knew I had to be at work the next morning. I ironed my suit, took another shower, ate a bowl of cereal and went back to sleep.

I woke up the next morning, and I was as hungover and dope sick as I've ever been. After throwing up for a half hour, I managed to get dressed and make a cup of coffee. It was early March by now and the weather had started to turn. It was a nice early spring morning and the fresh air made me feel somewhat human. I walked into the bank and moved toward my desk. As I got closer, I noticed Alex was sitting there.

"Hey Alex, what's going on, why are you at my desk?" I asked curiously.

Alex looked up at me with a look of absolute disbelief.

"Didn't Connie call you?" She asked.
"No, why?" I replied.

"Tommy, I'm sorry, but you don't work here anymore." Alex said, seeming confused by my disbelief.

Connie came behind me and asked if I could come downstairs to the break room with her. She looked at me with the concern of a loving parent and said,

"Tommy, we tried calling you after that first day you called in sick. You never answered your phone. You never called us, so we just assumed you weren't coming back. You are a smart young man. You have a lot of potential, but you also have a big problem, and you need to get yourself some help."

I looked at Connie with a straight face and said,

"Yes, you're right. My aunt is sick, and I really need to find some help taking care of her. Thank you for letting me go do that. I appreciate it. Do you have my last check?"

She looked at me with the same look my mother had been giving me for years. It was a look of defeat and sadness. She gave me my check and I left the bank. I was completely oblivious to the point she was trying to get across. You see, I hadn't been there in six weeks. I went through five thousand dollars in oxy, coke and booze, and never showed up to work. I didn't even remember calling in sick weeks earlier. I had no recollection of any phone calls. The fact that I would walk into a place of business after six weeks of not showing up, still thinking I had a job, shows the state of mind I was in. I took the money from the final paycheck I just received and stopped at the store. I bought a six pack of tall boys and drank three in the store to stop the shakes. I was about to hit the peak of dope sickness and I needed to get a fix.

As I was going into my pocket for a cigarette, I noticed a small round outline in the bottom of my jacket. It can't be. I tried desperately to wiggle the object through whatever hole it made its way through to get where it was. It was like a cruel joke. It could have been anything, but in my head, it was the pill I needed to get right. Finally having no other alternative, I chewed a hole in the bottom of the jacket of my favorite suit. Sure enough it was an OC40. I must have had it in my pocket the last time I wore the suit, and it somehow got stuck in the lining. Forty milligrams was nothing, but it was enough to ease some of the sickness. Five months prior I was making this walk home from my new job. I was happy. I felt like I was going to accomplish great things. I felt optimistic. In a matter of weeks, I threw that all away. I was out of a job and had no pills left. Only one thought dominated my brain.

How am I going to get more?

CHAPTER 19

Banished

Ilya hadn't picked up his phone in a few days and I was as sick as a dog. When he finally did pick up, he told me the heat was on at the pharmacy after they discovered hundreds of Oxycontin had gone missing. That wasn't good for anybody involved. He assured me it wouldn't blow back on him because the owner suspected someone else. He told me I would have to wait until everything died down before he could get me more. With no access to money or pills I became desperate. I was getting sicker by the day and I resorted to what I had been doing before I started working at the bank. My mother and aunt were in Pennsylvania for my six-week run, so they didn't see the disaster I had become in such a short time. They got home on a Friday morning and as I was helping them in with their stuff my aunt handed me her pocketbook to bring up to her apartment while she walked her dog. She let her guard down for a moment and that moment was all it took. I opened her bag when I got upstairs and there they were. Two bottles of OC80's and one hundred and twenty Perc 5/325's. I quickly opened all three bottles, taking ten each from the OC's and about twenty Percs. The brain is a crazy thing. When you're dope sick the simple thought of getting what you need makes the sickness subside and as soon as I saw those pills the symptoms went away. I quickly ran down the stairs and into my bathroom. I crushed and snorted two OC's followed by washing down five Percs with a warm beer that was sitting on my nightstand. Just like that I was back to stealing from my family.

The OC's and Percs were gone in two days and I was desperate. I was blowing up Ilya's phone and he wasn't answering. I felt that the story he told me was bullshit and he was avoiding me for some other reason. I called car service and went to the pharmacy he worked at. The last thing this guy needed was a strung-out junkie showing up and causing a scene with the supposed heat that he had on him. As soon as he saw me, he ran out from behind the counter. He took me outside and laid into me. He told me I could never show up there and that I was going to get us both locked up. He admitted that he made up the story because Yuri told him I was strung out and he shouldn't give me pills anymore. He commented on how bad I looked and asked me if I was getting high. I quickly shot that idea down, claiming I had the flu. I told him I had a big buyer, and I would need another five thousand worth of Oxy. I also told him I didn't have the money up front, but I would have it less than twenty-four hours after he floated me the pills. I had given Ilya close to ten grand over the last month, so he agreed to give me the pills on credit. The owner of the place was going on vacation the next day and he would be able to get me as much as he could without raising any red flags. He couldn't promise me the whole five thousand worth, but he would do his best. That was fine with me considering the whole story was bullshit and I never had any intention of giving Ilya the money for the pills anyway. A few hours later he called me and told me he could get me five bottles. Two bottles would be OC10's, two would be OC20's and one OC40. It wasn't the optimal result I was looking for, but it would suffice. I calculated that those pills would last about two weeks. Two weeks would give me enough time to figure out my next move. Two weeks came and went, and Ilya was blowing my phone up along with Yuri. The good thing is Ilya didn't know where I lived, and Yuri was so banged up the night he drove me home he didn't either. If I stayed in the neighborhood, I knew I wouldn't have to deal with them.

I woke up not really knowing what day it was. They all blend together after a while. I was out of pills, so I took five from my aunt. I snorted a couple and went to G's. We were smoking weed and drinking forties when it happened. G went to the bathroom and I saw the hundred dollars I spoke about in the beginning of my story. That was the hundred dollars that effectively ended my friendship with G. After I went home that night and did all the drugs, and drank all the booze I had left, I decided it was time for a break. I needed to get my shit together so I asked my cousin if he could come pick me up and take me to the house in Pennsylvania to dry out. He agreed to come the next weekend and get me. You would think a week wasn't enough to mess things up any more than they already were. You would be wrong. The only people who still tolerated me other than my own family were Patty, Joey, Kelly and their mother. One day I was in the house and I thought I was alone. I decided to rummage through drawers looking for money. I wasn't alone. Jim was there, and he heard me in the master bedroom. He had been living with the family for the last few years and he was in his room with his girlfriend. He told Joey what he saw and heard. I received a call a few hours later and Joey told me that I was no longer welcome in his house. In five days I had been banished from two homes that I spent ninety percent of my time in. I lost all my friends and I never felt more alone than I did in those following days. I told Ilya to go fuck himself and if he wanted his money he could come get it. I knew he had more to lose than me and chances were he would just cut his losses and move on.

My cousin came to pick me up the following Friday and I was a wreck. My aunt gave my cousin seven Percocet for his back because he was in legitimate pain. As soon as we walked in the door of the house in Jim Thorpe, I found, and took all seven pills. When he questioned me, I just denied it. I was the only other person for fifty miles so it couldn't be anybody else but me. I lied, I yelled, and he eventually gave up. I found every bottle of liquor I could find and drank it. He eventually poured whatever was left down the drain. In the middle of nowhere, with nobody around, my cousin opened the bedroom door and flipped me two joints, and told me to make them last because that's all I was getting for the rest of the week. I sat in that room alone for the next few days. I smoked the joints and took Benadryl to try and sleep. I was dope sick and I had the shakes. The depression was overwhelming, and I found myself crying most of the time I was awake. I lost all my friends. My family was disappointed and ashamed and I felt as hopeless as I ever had. I looked up on the wall and there it was. It was the shotgun my cousin had won in a raffle a few years earlier. I stared at it for what seemed to be an hour, then I stood on the bed and took it down from its perch. There is a stigma about suicide. People who take their own lives are labeled cowards and selfish. There was a time in my life when I thought the same way. My mind was changed that night. I sat on the edge of the bed with the gun pressed between the bottom of my chin and the floor. I thought about all the hurt I had caused people. I thought about the hurt I caused myself. I thought about a future without any of the people I loved in my life. The thoughts became overwhelming and I was weeping like a baby. I hated the way I was living, but it got to the point that I didn't know how to live any other way. I tried to squeeze the trigger, even asking God to give me the strength to do it. After a while I released the gun from my chin. I fell back on the bed, curled up in a fetal position, and cried myself to sleep.

I woke up the next morning and most of the physical withdrawal had subsided. I apologized to my cousin for taking the pills and we had a good talk. He was a maniac in his own right and had a lot of issues in life, but he was like my big brother. He, along with everyone else just wanted what was best for me. I wish I could say that I went home and straightened myself out after that awful night, but I can't. I didn't pull the trigger, but I was dead inside. All the thoughts that led me to that moment were still there and the only way I knew how to cope was the way I had been doing it for years, drinking and getting high.

CHAPTER 20

Auntie

Eileen Veronica Shirley was born January 13, 1936. She was one of four children. It was my Uncle Tommy, my Aunt Eileen and my Uncle Den. They were my mother's three older siblings. I loved all three, but my Aunt Eileen was my favorite. She was my godmother, and our relationship was special from day one. When I was four and five years old, the highlight of my life was sleeping over my aunt's house. At that time, her and my two cousins lived in a small apartment in Bay Ridge that my aunt referred to as the roach motel. I didn't care because if I was with my aunt, I was ok with the roaches. We would stay up late, eating ice cream and watching scary movies. She let me eat anything I wanted, and she ate anything I wanted. I mean anything. My favorite thing to do was play restaurant. I used to make these awful concoctions of everything she had in the refrigerator. I would pour salad dressing, pickle juice, orange juice, milk, butter and anything else I could find into a bowl. I would stir it up, bring it into the living room, and serve it to her on a little snack table. I would have a towel over my arm, and I would call her madam. She would look at me with a bit of horror on her face and ask me what it was. I used to tell her it was a special stew, compliments of the chef. I would stare at her and she would stare back. Eventually she would taste it. She would immediately get up and go to the bathroom to spit it out. Then she'd come back and tell me she was full. She would put the rest in the refrigerator and make sure to show my mother what I made her eat the next day. My mother would just shake her head and laugh.

When my aunt moved in to the second floor of my house when I was six, it was the happiest I had been up to that point in my life. Now, instead of going to the roach motel, I could just go upstairs whenever I wanted, spend time with her, and cook up more of my delicious recipes. We would spend hours together. On Saturday mornings I would go up and jump in bed with her. We would put on wrestling and watch the likes of Hulk Hogan, The Iron Sheik, Junkyard Dog and George the Animal Steel, beat the crap out of each other for two hours. When it was over, I would practice all the moves I just saw on my aunt. My cousin Stephanie would come in and scream, *"what the hell are you doing to her?"*, on a regular basis. My aunt would just say to leave me alone, I was just having fun. My aunt loved me and I loved her. Some, including her, would say I had her wrapped around my finger.

As I got older, the relationship only got stronger. She was more than my aunt. She was my friend. After my father left, she took it upon herself to be even more of an influence in my life. She felt that I needed someone, other than my mother, to confide in. She would be that person for me. There was nothing I couldn't tell her. As time went on, and I went off to college, she was the ying to my mother's yang. My aunt was a more street-smart version of my mother. When my mother had a hard time with me being away from home, my aunt was able to be the voice of reason. When my mother would voice concern over my behavior, my aunt would bluntly say;

"Dorothy, he drinks, he smokes, he sucks, he fucks. That's what kids his age do. For bloody sakes leave him alone already."

Looking back on it, my mother was one thousand percent right to be concerned, but my aunt, just like me, thought it was normal to do the things I was doing because that's what kids do. Anytime I was short on cash my aunt would make sure a two-hundred-dollar money order was in the mail a day later. When I got in trouble with Jimmy for being short for a few weeks, she took a bank loan out to pay my debt.

When I went into the psych ward, she was there to pick me up when I got out. She was there for me, through everything, no matter what. Of all the people I hurt when I was at my worst, my Aunt Eileen, my favorite person in the world, bore the brunt of it all.

One afternoon in the summer of 2002, my aunt and mother called me downstairs, telling me we needed to talk. At that stage of my life, we need to talk was almost always an intervention of some sort. Either that, or they found out I stole pills or money from them. When they finished talking to me, I found myself wishing it were one of those things. My aunt had been diagnosed with cancer. She had already beaten the disease twice, having most of her lung removed years earlier, and her breast removed long before I could remember. The breast cancer cells that had been dormant came back. I was devastated. I know I treated her terribly, but I loved her more than anyone on earth. Instead of being supportive and caring, I did what I always did. I made it all about me and used it as an excuse to get high.

After deservingly being removed from the lives of my friends, I spent most of 2003 by myself, in the house, only leaving to get alcohol or drugs. I continued to steal medication from my aunt who was growing sicker by the day. As the year went on, her trips to the hospital became more frequent, and her condition upon returning home became worse each time. One visit to the hospital stands out in my mind. I was out of oxy and starting to become sick. When I arrived at my aunt's room the nurse told me that they had just taken her down for a test and I was more than welcome to wait for her to come back. I sat in the chair next to her bed and started watching television. I became thirsty and turned to get the pitcher of water she had on the end table. That's when I noticed the little orange case she kept her pills in. I spent the better part of the last eighteen months hunting that thing down, and now there it was, right there for the taking. Everything in me told me to leave it alone, but I couldn't. I had to open it and see what was there. The inside of the case was divided into little triangular sections. When I opened it, each of the sections were filled with OC80's. My stomach tightened and I became flushed with adrenaline. I had done a lot of rotten things to this point. Most of it was to those closest to me, but if I did this, I would be crossing an unspeakable line. I put the case down and went into the bathroom. I threw water on my face and looked in the mirror. I hated what I was feeling, but the feeling was so powerful, I couldn't control it. I remember walking out of the bathroom. I looked at the case, then looked at the I.V. pole next to her bed, a bag of morphine hanging from it. I rationalized my choice by telling myself she would be fine without the pills because of the morphine. I walked over to the table and I took five pills out of each of the six sections. I put two in my mouth, chewed them, and washed them down with the water I had poured myself minutes earlier. I left the room and went to the diner around the corner from the hospital. I couldn't be there when she got back because I needed plausible deniability. If they realized the pills were missing and knew I was in the room, they would know it was me. If I showed up an hour after she got back, they would assume it was a random theft. If the nurse didn't mention I was there I would be good to go. It was a sick way to think, but by that point my mind was too sick to think any other way. I sat in that diner for an hour, drinking coffee, struggling with what I had just done. I would call her room every ten minutes to see if she had gotten back. Finally, after an hour she answered. She was so happy to hear from me. My mother had just gotten there, and she said they were about to watch Charmed, a show about witches, that she loved. I told her I just got off the train and I would be there in a few minutes. I went up to her room and sat with her, watching charmed for the next two hours, putting the guilt for what I had done earlier deep in the recesses of my brain.

She got out of the hospital a week later and her condition had grown worse. She couldn't make it up the stairs to her apartment, so we set her up in the basement. My Uncle Tom would come over every day and help. She had trouble getting up from the couch, so he built a wood support plank to give the couch more height. When she had to go to the bathroom, I would help her onto the commode next to the chair she would sit in. I would help her clean herself and put her back in her chair. She would thank me and cry, telling my mother how good I was to her, then, when she went to sleep, I would take her pills. Everyone was struggling to cope, but they were doing it. They were doing it because that's what family does for each other. I was doing it to get what I needed. My addiction came before anyone and anything.

She would be in and out of the hospital over the next few months. By now it was early 2004 and when she got home from her latest hospital stay, her legs were filled with fluid, and covered in sores. She had lost all her hair and was frail beyond words. She was a physical shell of the woman I once knew. Despite all this, she was still my auntie. She still argued with my mother over the same things they had been arguing over for years. She still cursed like a sailor and she still loved her soap operas and her Charmed. One afternoon she was having an especially difficult time getting up to go to the bathroom. She was in such severe pain she couldn't get out of the chair and wound up peeing on herself. We called the ambulance, and they came to take her for yet another hospital stay. I hugged her and told her I would see her later. I spent the rest of the day drinking and taking Oxy. My mother called that night and told me my aunt's condition had worsened and she would call when she had more news. Her last words to me on that call were "*please don't drink anymore tonight.*"

The door between the foyer and the living room swung open. It was my cousin telling me to get myself together because we had to go to the hospital. I must've passed out on the living room floor because I was wearing the same clothes from the day before. There were Budweiser cans all around me, and cigarette ashes all over the floor. I got up, finished the half can of beer that was left on the floor next to me, ate two OC's and jumped in the shower. The ride to the hospital was silent. My cousin didn't want me in her car any more than I wanted to be there. Our relationship was nonexistent since my behavior at the firm and being alone with her was very awkward. When we got to my aunts' room, I knew things weren't good. My mother and two uncles were there speaking with the doctor, and my uncle had tears in his eyes. I said my hellos and just looked at my aunt and cried. My mother came to hug me, and a look of disgust came on her face when she smelled the remanence of last night's activity seeping out of my pores. I knew that look. I had seen it on many faces over the years. I was almost numb to it by now. She patted my face lightly and told me to go sit with my aunt. I walked over to the bed and sat next to her. She looked peaceful. For the first time in a year she looked like she wasn't in pain. I held her hand and put my head next to hers. I told her how sorry I was for everything I did to her. I told her how much I loved her and that I didn't know what I was going to do without her. I imagine that in that moment, she saw the little boy that used to watch wrestling with her on Saturday mornings, not the person he had become. She looked at me with a tear coming from her eye, smiled, and simply said, *"I know darling, I know."* That was the first time she had called me darling in a long time. She turned her head away and looked at the ceiling. Her hand tightened on mine as she gasped her last breath. Her grip loosened, her breathing stopped, and she was gone. In the early morning hours of Friday, March 12, 2004, my Aunt Eileen passed away at age sixty-eight. She died surrounded by family, and as much as I didn't deserve it, I got to tell her how sorry I was for treating her how I did. Auntie, in life and in death, you always have been, and always will be, my guardian angel.

Rest In Peace
Eileen V. Shirley
1/13/36 – 3/12/2004

CHAPTER 21

365 Days Later

My aunts wake was held on the Sunday after she passed. People from the firm showed up for my cousin. I felt embarrassed facing them for the first time since my unceremonious departure from the company, but that's not what this night was about. They put their feelings about me aside and were very cordial. I even had a brief conversation with Bart outside where he seemed genuinely concerned about the way my life had played out. My friends also put their feelings aside and came to show their support, even offering a place to go and talk if needed. It showed that the situation had nothing to do with how they felt about me, but everything to do with the way I treated them and what I was doing to myself. Jeff came down with a few guys from Westchester to pay their respects. Jeff knew my aunt very well from our time together at Pace and his frequent visits to Brooklyn in the years since. Because of the distance between us, and my inability to do to him what I did to the rest of my friends, Jeff was one of the few that never stopped talking to me through my whole run of destruction. He didn't see the day-to-day progression, but that night he got a glimpse into what my life had become. A new episode of the Sopranos was airing that night. It was before DVR, so I sent Jeff to my house to put a tape in the VCR, record it, and get some beer so we could drink and watch the episode when the wake was over. When Jeff came back he had a look of concern on his face. When I asked if he set up the recording and got the beer, he replied that he indeed set up the recording, but he wasn't getting beer. He looked at me with a dead stare and said, *"dude, I think you have a problem."* I couldn't figure out where that was coming from, but when I got back to my house it all made sense. It had been six months since I slept in my bedroom. It wasn't because I didn't like the room or preferred the couch. It was because I couldn't find the bed. I would drink every night and stash the empties under, and behind the couch. My mother would often clean up and find my mess, putting it in a black garbage bag and displaying it in front of the television for me to see. To avoid this, I started disposing the empties in my own black bags and storing them in my bedroom. I had amassed so many black garbage bags of empty cans and bottles that you could barely open the door to walk in the room. When Jeff saw this, he realized how bad it had gotten and for the first time voiced his concerns. I shrugged it off and bought a six pack of twisted tea instead, watching the Sopranos later that night with Jeff, in awkward silence, and passing out on the living room floor.

My cousin Denis was there as well. He was my Uncle Den's son. He was six years younger than me and had the same issues I had. The only difference between me and him is he always got caught. He got locked up all the time and my uncle, being a retired cop, always got him out of it. We had grown close during the time my aunt was sick. At first it was because I had nobody else to hang out with, but as time went on, I liked spending time with him. When I went away to Pace we lost touch. When I came back to Brooklyn, I kept my distance, hearing all the stories about him fighting, stealing cars, and selling drugs, only seeing him at family functions. I was no better, and the truth was, he was a good kid who had a hard time growing up. My Uncle wasn't around much when my cousin was young having his own issues with the bottle and his mother was an absolute unadulterated psychopath, who made the home a very toxic place to live. She would call internal affairs on my uncle all the time, telling them he was selling drugs and beating her. She told my cousin from day one that he was the devil, and she wished he were never born. All this kid ever wanted was a normal family, and growing up, my aunt and mother tried to give him glimpses of that as much as they could. They would have cake for him on his birthday and give him presents only for his mother to stash them in a closet and never let him see them again. He didn't need the presents. All he needed was the family. He was always his happiest when he was with us, but he always had to go home. I was happy that we grew close, but the two of us together was a bad combination. One night he came to my house looking like he had just run there from Bay Ridge. When I asked what was wrong, he told me that the cops were watching him, and he had to stash his supply with me until the heat died down. He left me with eight ounces of weed and a bottle of ninety Vicodin 5/500. I asked if he wanted me to get rid of it for him and he said if I could, he would give me a cut. I wound up selling one ounce, smoking four, getting beat for three and eating all the Vicodin. He was livid about that for years after. It became a joke after a while with me always ending the argument saying it was his fault for leaving his drugs with me. It was a love hate relationship, but in the wake of my aunt's death, and the situation with my life, he was the only friend I had.

The following months were the darkest of my life. My aunt was gone and I missed her terribly. I also missed the supply of pills that her circumstances provided. Toward the end of my aunt's life, they used to keep the bulk of her medication in a lockbox in my cousin's bedroom. I would break into the box regularly, even after she died. One day, upon opening the box, I found a note from my cousin that said, *you should be ashamed of yourself*. I was, but at this point I didn't care anymore. With no access to Oxycontin, I had to find other ways of getting what I needed. Denis was able to get me Vicodin and Percocet from time to time, but not the amount I needed. I would go to Joe's Deli every morning to get my first six pack. I would frequently put it on credit, then pay at the end of the week with a bad check. Eventually Joe caught on to my game and threw me out of the store, telling me to never come back, another lifelong relationship, ruined by my addiction. With Joe's no longer an option, I started frequenting a deli on 11th Avenue, owned by an older Russian man and his son. His son was around my age and he was into a lot of crooked stuff. I spent a lot of time in the deli and we became friendly. I agreed to transport packages of weed, cocaine and money for him in exchange for a few bucks and free drugs. I was drinking, smoking and sniffing coke all day every day, but the thing I really wanted was opiates. At this point I didn't even care what kind, I just needed something to feed my need. The Russian eventually introduced me to a guy who would sell me his monthly prescription of Methadone and Klonipin pills. The combination of the two coupled with alcohol would send me into a daily blackout. I would lose days, sometimes weeks at a time, never knowing exactly what I did or who I did it with. One night I woke up at two o'clock in the morning, on my living room floor, covered in mussels and marinara sauce, with a big black lab sitting next to me eating out of the catering tin the food came in. The dog was owned by a guy that lived down the block, but to this day I still don't know where the food came from and how the dog wound up in the house with me. Another night I got a call from an inmate at Rikers Island. Apparently, I was partying with him the week before and agreed to move heroin for him while he was in jail, yet another night I have no recollection of. This went on for a few months until one day when I went to the deli to get my beer and pick up whatever package I was to deliver. To my surprise the deli was closed. I went back later that day and again the next, but it was still closed. The deli, under that owner, never opened back up. I never saw the Russian again and just like that my source of money and drugs disappeared. As I was contemplating my next move, in stepped Geno.

Geno lived down the block from me. He was the older kid to the older kids when I was growing up. Geno was out of his mind. He was in and out of jail his whole life and was known to have his own issues with drugs. All that being said, he was the most likable drug addict I ever knew. Everyone in the neighborhood loved him. He was always polite and quick to help anyone in need. One of his schemes was gathering shopping lists from the women in the neighborhood. He would take the list to the local Pathmark and stick cuts of meat down his pants and in his jacket. He would then sell the meat to the women at half price. It was a win win for everybody except Pathmark. His other go to was driving around in a van, collecting stuff people had put out with the trash. He would do this every night then sell the stuff the next day out of his yard. There were always people lined up to see what treasures Geno had uncovered the night before, and it became a nice little racket for him. I started hanging out with Geno because he was the only person left in the neighborhood that would talk to me, and, because he had a good connection for cocaine. Tiny was a Puerto Rican kid from Sunset Park that Geno had met at his parole office. I first started using him through Geno until one night when Geno got pinched buying cocaine for me. He took the collar and didn't say a word. When he got out a few days later I thanked him and asked him if he happened to have my two hundred dollars, to which he replied," *Figgy, don't push your luck.*" After that night I met with Tiny myself.

Geno didn't like to snort cocaine. He thought it was a waste. What he loved to do was smoke it. He would frequently ask if I wanted to try it, but I would always refuse. There weren't many lines I hadn't crossed yet and that was one of them. One day I called Tiny and asked him for a fifty bag of the soft. The soft was powder and the hard was crack or base. He told me he was on his reup and it would be a few hours before he could get to me. He told me he had dropped off the soft to Geno earlier that morning so I should call him and see if he had any. I thought it was strange because Geno never got the soft. When I went down to Geno's house and asked him if he had any coke, he said yes and motioned to the stove. He was making his own crack. My stomach tightened and the adrenaline started flowing through my body, much like the first time I tried cocaine, the first time I took Oxycontin and the night in my aunt's hospital room. Anytime I was presented with a choice that I knew would take me to another level of addiction I got those feelings. This was another one of those times. Everything that was sensible and good in me told me this was a line I shouldn't cross, but like those other times, I crossed it anyway. He didn't have a pipe handy, so he put a fragment of one of the rocks on a piece of tin foil. He handed me a lighter, the tube of a Bic pen, and instructed me on what to do. With the tube in my mouth, I heated the bottom of the foil and watched the rock start to bubble. As the smoke started to rise, I leaned the tube over the foil and inhaled the smoke into my lungs. I held it for ten seconds and exhaled. A rush of euphoria overtook my body and I smiled at Geno, who was nodding in approval. I immediately called Tiny and told him to change my order from the soft to the hard. When I went home, I was short on cash, so I grabbed two bags of empty cans that I had stored in my bedroom. I went up to Pathmark and exchanged them for cash. Just like that, everything the guy said to me in the psych ward two years earlier came true. I never stopped thinking how I was thinking, so I never stopped doing what I was doing, now two years later I was trading cans for crack money. His story was now mine.

The days, weeks and months ahead grew darker. Me and Geno came up with another scheme to get drugs. He called me down to his house and showed me a prescription pad he stole from his doctor's office. I immediately put the plan together in my head. I knew how to write a prescription from years of filling them myself. The plan was to write myself a script for ninety pills. I would cash the script and split the pills with Geno. He would trade his for crack while I would get high on mine. It had to be Vicodin, which back then was a schedule III narcotic. Percocet was a schedule II which needed a whole different prescription. I would wait until the evening when I knew the doctor's office was closed, that way the pharmacy couldn't call to confirm the validity of the script. I would clean myself up and put on my blue suit. I needed to look like I was a somewhat respectable human being. I would only use big chain pharmacies and never use two in the same area more than once in the same month. Following these steps would increase the chances of succeeding while lessening the chances of me getting caught. It was an anxiety filled, nerve-wracking process, but it always went off without a hitch. I did this about thirty times over the next two months. As with anything else, the more I had, the more I used. When the pad ran out of sheets, I had once again developed a physical habit. One night I was at Geno's and I was visibly sick. He asked me what was wrong and I told him it was withdrawal from the Vicodin. I asked of he could get me anything to help me out. He made a few calls and told me the only thing he could get was heroin. It was the last line. That was the only thing I hadn't graduated to, but at this point I didn't even try to stop myself. I immediately said yes and an hour later I had a bundle of heroin in my hand. I grabbed two forty ounces of Budweiser and went back to my house.

It was October 16, 2004. I remember this for two reasons. The first being that it was Joeys birthday. I remember seeing them sitting on his porch getting ready to go out and celebrate. I wished him a happy birthday as I walked by and he just nodded and said thanks. The second reason was that it was the 2004 NLCS. The one thing I still got some joy out of was watching sports, especially playoff baseball. There was something about the whole atmosphere of a baseball stadium in October that gave me a sense of comfort. Roger Clemens was pitching for the Astros that night and I was looking forward to watching. When I got home I knew I needed to get well if I was going to enjoy this game. I went into my bathroom and took the bundle of heroin out of my pocket. I had never done heroin before and I didn't know how much I should do. I emptied two of the glass line baggies onto the counter and snorted them. I didn't feel much, so I did another. That's when it hit me, just like the night I took my first Oxycontin. The rush, the warmth and the euphoria washed over me, and all was right with the world. I threw up a few times, then went to my living room and watched the game while sipping on my forties. Clemens threw a gem and the Astros won the game. That bundle lasted into the next day before I got another, then another, then another. Within a month I was snorting two bundles of heroin a day. Finally, one afternoon I went to Geno's looking for more. Geno took one look at me, motioned his hands like he was wiping them clean and said,

"Figgy, you're out of control. I can't get that for you anymore."

Geno, the guy who everyone looked at and said don't become like him, just told me that I was out of control. What the fuck kind of twilight zone episode was I in? That was the day I had no more fingers to point. That was the day I realized that I was now the guy that parents would look at and say, *don't become like that guy.* The next few months were out of control. Tiny hooked me up with a heroin dealer, but he was unreliable. I was smoking two hundred dollars' worth of crack and drinking a liter of vodka every day. To get my opiate fix, I would punch the brick wall in my back yard or beat myself in the shoulders and knees with a baseball. When I was sufficiently swelled and bruised, I would go to the emergency room and make up a story of how I sustained my injuries. More often than not they would prescribe me Vicodin or Percocet. After a while they started to catch on to my game and I was flagged as a drug seeker by three local hospitals. One night, out of money and out of options, Tiny offered to trade me five hundred dollars worth of crack for my watch. My watch was the only nice thing I had left. My mother bought it for me the Christmas before my aunt died and I refused to trade it for drugs. A week later I sold it to him for twenty dollars of crack and ten Percocet.

It was March of 2005. It was almost a year since my aunt died and I was worse now than at any time she was alive. I started thinking of the words I said to her in her final moments and how little they would mean if I continued living the way I was living. I stopped smoking crack on March 1st. I had been off heroin for a few months already, and with the hospitals cutting me off, the ten Percocet from Tiny were that last opiates I had taken. I cut my drinking down to a couple of beers a day and stopped smoking weed. At the dinner table on March 11th, I told my mother I was considering getting clean for good. She was very happy to hear but skeptical at the same time. I asked her for twenty dollars to get pills for my heartburn. That is what I had every intention of getting. She reluctantly gave me the money and I walked up to Pathmark to get some Pepcid. As I was searching for the medication I came across a box of Coricidin. Coricidin is a cold medicine that contains Dextromorphan. I saw a dateline special a few weeks earlier about it and if taken in a high enough dose, it produces a psychedelic high. I couldn't resist and I bought a box. The weeks of tapering my drug use and drinking were out the window. The words I said to my mother minutes earlier meant nothing. I went home and took half the box. An hour later I was flying. The high was out of control and it scared me. Out of my mind on cold medicine, my mother called me into her room. She took one look at my eyes and demanded to know what I had taken. I denied being high, even blowing in her face to show my breath didn't smell like alcohol. She wasn't buying it and she spoke in a voice I had never heard before. She was finally done. All the years of me killing myself slowly right in front of her came to a boiling point. I knew she was about to throw me out. The one person I had left was about to give up. I couldn't blame her. I had given up on myself long before that. In that moment I saw the reflection of myself in the mirror. I saw what I had been trying so hard to avoid seeing the last few years. I could hardly recognize myself. I looked dirty, my face was bloated and yellow tinted. My eyes were outlined by dark circles and there was nothing behind them. There was no feeling and no hope. I saw complete defeat. It was in that moment I realized that if I didn't change my life, not only would I lose the only support I had left, I was going to die. I looked at my mother and told her I was done. I asked her to call my cousin and meet me in the living room. I went on to tell them everything I had done over the last few years. I told them I wanted help and that I was truly ready to change my life. They looked at me in stunned silence. It was a lot to take in, and I don't blame them if they didn't believe a word I said to them that night because I said the words a hundred times before. What they didn't know, what nobody could know except myself, was that this time was different. I knew I was ready. By that time the clock struck past midnight and it was March 12th and it was a year since my aunt had passed away. I looked at my mother and cousin and said that this day would be a good day from now on. This day would be my new beginning. March 12, 2005 would now be the start of my second chance at life.

CHAPTER 22

A New Beginning

When I woke up Sunday morning I felt different. The first thought upon waking over the last few years had always been where I was going to get my next drink or my next high. Today it wasn't there. My mother set up a memorial mass for the anniversary of my aunt's death. We were meeting my Uncle Tom and Aunt Joyce at St. Rosalia's Church on 14th Avenue at nine o'clock. I got dressed and relaxed on the couch with a cup of green tea while I waited for my mother and cousin. We went to the mass and had breakfast afterwards at a local diner. It was the first time in a long time I wasn't embarrassed to sit with my family. I know it had only been less than twelve hours since I got high, but it was the feeling inside that let me be comfortable in that setting. I wanted to tell my aunt and uncle of my decision to change my life. I wanted to tell anyone who would listen, but I realized nobody wanted to hear words. They wanted to see change.

After breakfast we went home and I spent the rest of the day on the computer looking up outpatient treatment programs and twelve step meetings in the area. The following day I would set forth on a mission to change my life. That night I took an early shower, shaved, and cut my hair. I settled into bed and started watching an episode of intervention. The episode hit home with me and I found myself crying uncontrollably. I found myself crying a lot in those early days. I would come to find out, those were my emotions coming back to life. I was suppressing everything for so long that I wasn't used to feeling the broad spectrum of feelings a human has when not on drugs. The only two I had the last few years were elation and misery, misery being the dominant one for much of that time.

Monday morning I woke up at eight o'clock. I made myself a cup of coffee and got on the phone. I called an outpatient rehab in Bay Ridge named Bridge Back to Life. It was a catchy name, and the only one I could remember not getting thrown out of a few years earlier. I answered a bunch of questions and set up an appointment to meet with a counselor the next morning. Now it was time for a meeting. The first one I had circled was being held at one of the local hospitals at eleven o'clock. I found it ironic I was going to a place I had been flagged by as a drug seeker just a month earlier for my first meeting. I started walking, and for the first time in years, I noticed things like the sun on my face and the smell in the air. I saw the color of the sky and realized I couldn't remember the last time I walked with my head up. That morning it felt good to be alive. When I got to the hospital, I couldn't find the meeting. I eventually asked a hospital employee who told me the meeting had closed a month earlier. Ordinarily, a setback like that would send me into a tailspin and I would go to the nearest deli, buy beer and start looking for drugs shortly after, but not today. I went home, ate lunch and found the next meeting on the schedule. It was at seven o'clock that night in Bay Ridge and I couldn't wait to go. The only problem was that it was only one o'clock. What was I going to do for the next six hours to occupy my mind?

As I was sitting on the couch watching an episode of NYPD Blue, I remembered the book the man in the psych ward had given me three years earlier. I went into my room and into the duffle bag I had thrown the book in minutes after he gave it to me. When I opened it, the inside cover had the date March 13, 1984, his first name and his last initial, written in the top left corner. When I saw that my mind was instantly put at ease. What are the chances that I would open that book three years after it was given to me, and the date inside would be twenty-one years to the date it was given to him? I had no idea what a higher power truly meant at that time, but it was surely a sign that one was working in my life. I spent the next three hours reading the stories in that book and I related to all of them. I remembered an episode of the Sopranos where Christopher comes back from rehab. He's talking to Tony and they are speaking about the twelve steps. He talks about the one where you go around making amends to people for all the shitty things you did to them over the years, to which Tony replies, maybe you should skip that one. I had a few more hours to kill, so I decided to write letters to all my friends on the block that I had wronged over the years. I wrote for two hours, then walked to each house and presented these letters. Some face to face and some I just left in the mailboxes. I explained that I knew they couldn't forgive me in that moment, but that I was trying to do the right thing now, and maybe in time, they could find it in them to accept my sincere apologies. Some were accepted graciously, some not, but writing them kept me out of my own head for a few hours, and by the time I was finished, it was time to head to the meeting.

When I walked up to the Church entrance there were a few people standing outside smoking cigarettes. I walked up and asked if I was in the right place. One of them looked at me and asked,

> *"You tired of getting drunk and high?"*
> *"Yes."* I replied.
> *"Then you're in the right place my friend. Welcome. My name is Vinny."*

I immediately felt comfortable. Vinny was right out of central casting for a neighborhood Italian guy. He was nicknamed Baba just for that reason. Me and Vinny would have many heart to heart talks over the next few years. When I walked down the stairs into the meeting, I was nervous. As comfortable as Vinny made me feel, I was still walking into the unknown. The feelings of insecurity that I had as a kid never went away, they were just masked by alcohol and drugs. Now, I would have to meet all new people and navigate a whole new life without that crutch. I became very overwhelmed in that moment and almost turned around and left. Just then, I heard my name being called. How does anyone know me? This isn't my neighborhood and its my first time here. I looked in the direction of the voice and there he was. Kyle was my neighbor. He rented the second floor apartment in the house next door to me and I used to sell weed to his roommate. When I would sit out on my porch every night getting high he would sit and talk to me, but he would never smoke. One night he came home, hyped up and ready to party. He had a twelve pack of Heineken and asked if I knew where to get coke. We wound up drinking and getting high for two days. After that he was weird around me. He didn't sit out and talk to me anymore, and his hellos became less friendly, eventually, he stopped saying hello at all. Sure, it was strange, but I was so caught up in my own shit, I never thought too much of it. He went on to explain to me that up until that night he had been sober for a little over two years. His girlfriend broke up with him and that led him to start drinking. That two-day binge he had with me was a relapse. A day later he started going back to meetings and now he was sober six months. He apologized for being cold towards me but explained that he had to stay away from me. People, places and things is a commonly used phrase in recovery. It means that you need to stay away from the people you got high with, the places you got high in and the things that trigger you in the first place. I had become one of those people to Kyle. I completely understood what he meant and told him he didn't need to apologize. If anything, I was the one who should feel guilty. He assured me it had nothing to do with me. If it wasn't me, it would've been someone else he got high with that night. He was happy to see me there and I was happy to see him. That familiar face and ten-minute conversation kept me from leaving my first meeting.

When the meeting started, a man sat in front of the room and read a bunch of stuff telling what the program was about. He read a list of people's names and how many years they were sober, then he asked if anyone with less than a year wanted to introduce themselves. My stomach tightened and I became flushed with adrenaline. There was that feeling again. I was presented with a choice, only this time the choice would take me in another direction. Once I put it out there I couldn't take it back. Once I said those words, I would have to own them and act on them. Person after person said their name and how long they had. When the man leading the meeting asked if there was anyone else, I raised my hand.

"My name is Tommy, I'm an alcoholic and an addict. I have two days."

My words were met with a huge round of applause. Kyle turned and gave me a fist bump. The guy behind me patted me on the back and welcomed me. The feeling of relief I felt in that moment was indescribable. It was like a five-hundred-pound weight had been taken off my shoulders. It was finally out there and now I could begin to heal. The rest of the meeting was a blur. The speaker told his story for twenty minutes and people made comments around the room. I can't remember what was said or who said it. What I do remember is I loved it. When the meeting was over, person after person came up to me and shook my hand. They welcomed me and told me if I kept coming back a day at a time, things would get better. A few days before, I thought my life was over. At twenty-nine years old I thought it was too late to turn things around and I felt completely hopeless. I don't know exactly what happened that night, but after meeting those people and hearing their words, I no longer felt hopeless. If I could do what they did, maybe there was a chance the things would be ok.

CHAPTER 23

The Fresh

I started my outpatient program the next morning at nine o'clock. My counselor was a Hasidic Jewish man named Rich. During my intake interview he started reading a list of substances, asking me if I used them or not. Halfway through the list I told him it would be a lot quicker asking me what I hadn't done. He got a laugh out of my comment and called me a wiseass, but then he turned all business. He bluntly told me that I was lucky to be alive and if I had any chance going forward, I would have to change everything. If anyone said that to me a week earlier, I would've told them to go fuck themselves, then went and got high. On this day I was all ears. Changing everything seems like a herculean task, but I was so tired of living the way I was living, I was ready to do anything. If that meant listening to an old Jewish guy in an office, or a bunch of people in a church basement, then so be it, nothing was going to stop me from turning things around. I would go to the program four days a week. Three days would be in a group setting and one day would be a one on one with Rich. The one on ones were my favorite. When Rich saw how dedicated I was to the program he took a liking to me, and the one on ones, while serious and painful at times, became the best part of my week. He would teach me about Jewish culture in between me telling him of all my misdeeds over the years. *"You get out what you put in."* he would say to me in his high-pitched voice. I bought in one hundred percent. I was in that program for six months, and I can honestly say I learned more in there than I did in five years in college.

On that first day, Rich stressed the importance of meetings. He told me the four hours I spent there were great, but I needed support outside of that place. I was happy to hear that because the one meeting I went to the night before was great. I hadn't felt that good about myself since I was fifteen years old. I was all about meetings and I couldn't wait to get to my next one. One thing suggested early on in twelve step meetings is to get a home group and a commitment. A home group is exactly what it says. It is your home. A commitment gives you a responsibility to be there. The doors need to be opened, the chairs need to be set up, and the coffee needs to be made. God forbid the coffee isn't ready when the first old timer walks through the door. You get to know people and they get to know you. If you're off, people will notice. If you don't show up, people will call. It becomes like a family. I had been so irresponsible and so alone for such a long time that a homegroup sounded like something I really needed. Ironically enough, on St. Patrick's Day 2005, one of the biggest drinking days of the year, I would find mine.

I was clean and sober for five days now, and while that doesn't seem like much, it was like a lifetime for me. I couldn't go five minutes without being drunk, being high, or obsessing about the two. I found a meeting close to home. I had been taking the bus to Bay Ridge since Monday, so being able to walk to a meeting in the neighborhood was a nice treat. The walk that Thursday night, to that church basement in Dyker Heights, would change my life for the better in more ways than I could ever imagine. It was six thirty when I walked up to the address. For a minute I didn't think I was in the right place. There were no people outside smoking cigarettes and the place seemed very quiet. All the lights in the building were off and the doors were locked. I pulled the meeting list out of my pocket and realized the meeting wasn't until seven thirty. How was I going to kill an hour? For a moment I thought about going home and calling it a night. Two nights earlier, I walked all over Brooklyn. While walking to 94th Street and 4th Avenue, I ran into my Aunt Grace. We talked for a half hour and missed the meeting. I looked at my list and saw there was a meeting on 84th street and 18th avenue, which is a mission from Bay Ridge. I got there on time, only to find out the meeting time had been moved up an hour and the list hadn't been updated. I went home that night and saw Kyle outside his house. I was upset that I didn't make a meeting, and he must have seen the disappointment on my face. When I told him what happened, he assured me that the effort I put in that night, more than made up for my bad timing and faulty meeting list. I could've easily used that same logic standing outside those locked doors, to go home and watch tv, telling myself I put the effort in and that's all that mattered, but I didn't. If I really wanted this, I had to be committed to it. I sat on the small step in front of the door, lit a cigarette and waited. About twenty minutes later a man walked up.

> *"Hey kid, what's going on?"* He said in a high pitched, raspy voice.
> *"Nothing much. I misread the meeting list and got here early."*
> I replied.
> *"Good, you can help me with the chairs, I'm Steve."* He said.
> Almost elated that he didn't have to do it himself.
> *"Nice to meet you Steve, I'm Tommy."*

We went downstairs and he told me to set the chairs up in a circle while he made the coffee. We got to talking. I told him part of my story and he told me some of his. He had two years at the time and when I told him I had five days he shook his head and commented that I must still be hurting. Truthfully, I felt great. It wasn't until months later that people would tell me how bad I looked in my first few weeks. It made sense. I just came off a twelve-year run of insanity. Five days wasn't going to make the outside look good, but inside, I was thrilled to be alive. People started rolling in around seven-fifteen. I recognized a few of them from the two meetings I had been to in Bay Ridge earlier that week. They remembered my name and told me they were happy to see me again. One even told me my day count. These people were for real. They genuinely seemed to care, and that made me feel good. Just then it felt like someone hit me in the back with a shovel. I turned around and looked in disbelief. Why was this guy, that I didn't know, smashing me in the back and laughing? It was in that moment that he grabbed me and gave me a big bear hug. I didn't know what was going on at this point. He was dressed in a denim jacket, psychedelic tie dye t-shirt, perfectly ripped jeans and motorcycle boots, looking like an extra from a Grateful Dead movie, topped off with a big 1970's style moustache and red bandana tied tightly around his head. He was loud, spoke fast and was obviously very friendly. I heard Steve's voice in the background.

"Put the kid down Dougie. You're going to scare him away." He let go of me and finally took a minute to introduce himself.
"Hey kid, I'm Dougie. Are you new?"
"Yea man, I have five days."
"Alright, five days is great. Welcome."

Just like that he picked me up again and gave me another bear hug. After about fifteen seconds he put me down and I took my seat in the circle. Just like the other meetings, the leader gave the rundown about the programs purpose and read a list of upcoming sober anniversaries. When he was finished the lights shut. He put a candle on the floor in the center of the room and sat back down. This night was getting stranger by the minute. First, I had pseudo-Jerry Garcia manhandling me for ten minutes, now we're shutting lights and lighting candles. I was about to leave when the leader introduced the speaker. Sure, enough it was Dougie. He spoke for twenty minutes. I was glad the lights were off, because when he was done I had tears in my eyes. He had been working as a drug counselor when the stress of the job coupled with him not going to meetings caused him to relapse on Xanax after eighteen years of sobriety. His wife passed away a few years earlier and he was the widowed parent of a young daughter. He was now a few years back sober, and with all the turmoil in his life he was still grateful and happy. He started this meeting years earlier to give people freedom to talk about whatever they wanted. Back then more so that today, it was frowned upon to speak of drugs in AA and vice versa. This meeting was there to speak on both. Dougie's story touched me and it inspired me to share that night. I went on too long, but nobody stopped me. I unloaded years of hurt, guilt, anger and sadness onto Dougie and the rest of the people in that room. When it was done and the lights went on, they didn't look at me differently, they didn't judge me, they didn't laugh. They embraced me and told me they did the same things I did. They made me feel a part of. They made me feel at home. As we were leaving, Steve told me to meet him back there at six thirty the next night. There was a seven fifteen meeting and he needed help with the chairs. There was also a business meeting beforehand where I would be able to join the group. The room I will refer to as the Fresh, Dougie, and people like him, would become the foundation my recovery would be built on.

CHAPTER 24

A Celebration

The days turned to weeks and the weeks turned to months. I met so many people in those first ninety days, I could barely remember all their names. Aside from Dougie, there was Vinny Baba, who I met that first night. There was Little Joey and his brother Ash, who would become my first sponsor. There was Stevie Mags who would pick me up every Saturday morning to get bagels for the big meeting in Bay Ridge. There was Kevin the Cop, who was a retired detective, and one of the nicest guys I ever met. Aside from helping newcomers like myself, he would spend his time volunteering at soup kitchens feeding the homeless. Last, but not least, was Betty. Betty was a very intimidating looking woman. She was small in stature, but she had that, *I will fuck you up if you say the wrong thing, Brooklyn look about her.* I would see her all the time at meetings but was always afraid to say hello. One night at a meeting, Little Joey told me that Betty was sixty-three years old. I didn't believe him. There was no way she was that old. After a lot of convincing, and me still being a gullible newcomer, I thought what better way to break the ice then tell her how great she looked for her age. Long story short, Betty was in her forties. I swear she was about to punch me in the face when Little Joey came from behind me laughing hysterically. He must've done this often because Betty cursed at him and chased him away. After apologizing to Betty for my idiotic assumption, she just looked at me and told me it was fine. She realized I was trying to compliment her and she appreciated it. We smoked a cigarette together, and from that moment on, me and Betty became great friends. After a while, her and Dougie would call me the son they never had, and I would refer to him as dad, and her as Momma Betty. Those are just a few of the many that would take me under their wing and show me how to navigate life as a productive member of society.

A productive member of society needs a job. I hadn't worked in two years and I didn't have a cent to my name. Aside from the obvious financial situation, I just needed something to make me feel useful. I was a twenty-nine-year-old man. In the early days of sobriety my mother used to give me money for the bus and a dollar to put in the basket at the meeting. If it weren't for her letting me live in her home, I would've been in the street a long time before. Guys would tell me to concentrate on my sobriety, but I needed to do something. Work wasn't going to find me, so I needed to find it. I had huge holes in my resume between 2000 and 2005. I only worked for a little over two years combined in those five, and I didn't exactly leave either job on the highest of notes. I didn't need a career, I just needed something to hold me over until I figured out what I wanted to do with my life. I looked in the local paper and saw an ad. It was for a company called Imperial Steam Cleaning. All I read was flexible hours, no experience and good pay. I called immediately and set up an interview for the next day. When I walked in the office there were ten guys there. I sat down in the group and eagerly waited to be called upon for my interview. That's not what happened. After a few minutes of waiting a man walked in the door. He introduced himself as Chet and he spoke like an extra from Goodfellas. He explained what the company did, what the pay and hours would be, and what he expected from us. When he was done, eight people got up and left. Me and a guy named Chino were the only two that remained. Chet looked at both of us and said in his overdone Brooklyn street guy accent,

"Looks like yous two guys got the job. See yous tomorrow night at nine."

Imperial cleaned oven exhaust systems for restaurants. Chet opened the company a few months before and had accounts all over the tri state area. He had a nice little business. His clients included TGIF, McDonald's, Popeyes, White Castle, Burger King, and various privately owned establishments. The job was gross, and the hours were awful, but the pay was good, and it made me feel human. I was able to buy some new clothes, give my mother money for the house, play golf with Ash and Kevin the Cop, and go out for coffee after meetings with Doug, Betty and the rest of the crew from the Fresh. After six months Chet made me a "Captain", and I led my own team of workers. In the fall of 2005, Chet wound up in rehab for his own drinking issues, and I ran his company while he was away. When he got back, he was impossible to deal with. He started to lose a lot of his clients and was firing anyone who didn't see eye to eye with him. I learned in recovery that it's ok to walk away from toxic situations that will negatively impact your life. Chet, and Imperial, were a toxic situation, and after ten months of working there, I decided it was in my best interest to leave the company. That job showed me that it didn't matter what you did for a living, if you did it with pride, and put your all into it, you can succeed at whatever you do.

Life was going great. A lot of my friends saw the improvement in me and started talking to me again. In June of 2005 I was invited to, and able to attend Joey's wedding. It was the first wedding I attended sober since I was a little kid, and I had a great time. I was asked to be in Mikey's bridal party later that year, and I was talking to Patty and the other Joey again on a regular basis. I graduated my outpatient program, I was chairing the Friday night meeting at the Fresh every week, and just like that it was March 12, 2006 and I was sober for one year. So much had changed in such a short time. I celebrated at the Fresh on St. Patrick's Day 2006, exactly one year after I made it my home and meeting was packed. One year is a big deal, and people from all the meetings that I attended over that year came to celebrate with me. In the front row was my cousin Stephanie, my mother, my Aunt Joyce, Tina (Joey, Patty and Kelly's mother), Joey and his wife Pam, Mikey and his wife Danielle, Ralph and Kelly, and my Aunts friend Georgina. Her and my aunt worked together in the hospital in the 80's and 90's. They remained friends, and she would come to the house to take care of my aunt in her final days. Every day at noon, without fail, she would come into my living room, sit next to me, and pray. In those moments, the last thing I wanted was a pastor getting in the way of me getting my load on, and I let her know it every time, but that didn't stop her. She would tell me that one day I would find the light and I would be ok. Now two years later, her prayers had come to fruition. It was hands down the proudest moment of my life.

After the leader opened the meeting, Dougie went up to present me with my one year coin. I went up to the front of the room and he gave me a hug, much like the one he gave me on that first night a year earlier. When I caught my breath and faced the room full of people, my eyes quickly focused in on the front row. It was a collection of the people that I hurt the most. The fact they were there said a lot about them, and it said a lot about the change I had made. It was overwhelming and when I tried to speak, I couldn't. My life flashed quickly before me and a wide array of emotions overtook my mind. I thought of all the mistakes I made, I thought of all the people I hurt and the times I wanted to die. I thought about how far I had come, and how good life could be if I stayed on this path. Finally, I thought how proud my aunt must be looking down on this moment. I broke down and cried for a solid three minutes straight. Every time I tried to talk, the tears came again. I finally got it under control, only to see many of the people in the room, fighting to hold back tears of their own. I thanked my mother and cousin for never giving up on me. I thanked my friends for letting me back in their lives, and I thanked the people in that room who welcomed me into their world and showed me a better way to live. For years I didn't think I could live without alcohol and drugs. Now I don't know how I ever lived with them. We went out to dinner after the meeting. My family and friends mingled and traded stories about the old me and the new. Dougie pulled me aside when it was all over and told me he was proud of me. I thanked him for his support and friendship and we hugged. As he was leaving, he turned to me and said,

> *"Hey son, you know what comes after a year?"*
> *"No Dougie. What comes after a year?"*
> *"A year and a day kid, a year and a day. See you in the morning."*

CHAPTER 25

One of The Strongest

During the time between the firm and the bank, my mother would always be on my case about taking civil service exams. I would buy the local paper, find what tests were being given, and give her a rundown of the ones I was planning on taking. She would give me money to pay for them, and I would use that money to buy drugs. On the day of the exams, I would leave the house early in the morning, drink all day, then come home and tell her how great I did. List after list would come out and I was obviously never on one. When she would ask why, I would just shrug my shoulders and claim to have no idea why I didn't pass the test. After a dozen or so times, she caught on to my game and stopped giving me money for them. On an early Saturday morning in the spring of 2003, as I was laying in bed, hungover from the night before, my mother came storming into my room. She started yelling at me to get up and meet her in the car in a half hour. When I made excuses not to go along with her plan, she threatened me with eviction. That was different. I had gotten many lectures over the years, but that was the first time I was threatened with being thrown out in the street. I got up, got dressed, sniffed a few OC's to get myself somewhat well, and met her in the car. She got on the Belt Parkway and drove for about forty minutes. She eventually got off and navigated her way through the streets of East New York, Brooklyn. She pulled up in front of Franklin K. Lane High School on Jamaica Avenue and handed me two pencils and an admittance card. It was the test for the New York City Department of Sanitation. She secretly applied for me because she knew I couldn't be trusted to do it myself. She drove me there because I couldn't be trusted to get there myself. She was going to do everything in her power to make sure I took that test. I looked at her like she was crazy. I was too good for this. A cop, yes, a fireman, yes, a paramedic, no problem, but a garbage man, there was no way. I was two weeks removed from having a shotgun under my chin, wanting to end my life because of how bad it had gotten. I had nobody and nothing in my life, yet in my convoluted brain, picking up garbage was beneath me. She told me to go in the building, take the test and take it seriously. She would wait outside for the duration of the exam. If I tried leaving, she would leave me there and I would be on my own from that day on. After a long back and forth I finally gave in. Three years later, my mother's persistence and my reluctant decision to walk in that building to take that test, would turn out to be one of the best decisions I ever made, and the answer to both of our prayers.

After I left Chet and Imperial, I was once again unemployed. I still had some money to hold me for a while, but I didn't want to get stagnant. Life was going well, and I didn't want anything to set me back. I would speak to people at meetings and voice my concerns. One afternoon I was sitting with Stevie Mags on his porch smoking a cigar. I told him I felt useless again and that if I didn't find a job soon I didn't know what I was going to do. It was the beginning of August and it had been a year since I was called by the Sanitation Department for my medical exam. I passed all the tests and got my CDL license which was a requirement of the job, yet a year later I still hadn't heard anything back from them. He looked at me and told me to relax. He told me to keep doing the next right thing, keep praying, and eventually good things would happen. He also told me to eat a chocolate bar. Stevie could never be totally serious, so after any heartfelt advice he ever gave me, he would always follow it up with something silly that had nothing to do with the topic at hand. I nodded my head and smiled.

I thanked him for his encouraging words, but inside, I was starting to feel somewhat hopeless. I grabbed a slice of pizza and headed home to watch the Met game. On the walk home Stevie's words echoed in my head and I asked God for help. When I walked in the door the phone rang, I picked it up and the voice on the other end said,

"Is this Thomas Figlioli?"
"Yes it is." I replied.
"Thomas, this is Mr. Jones from the Department of Sanitation. We would like you to come in Monday at 8:00AM for final processing."

I had been waiting on that call for a year. My prayer was answered. I used to make fun of Patty for taking the job years earlier. I looked down on it, but that had everything to do with me and the disillusioned way I used to think. I now saw the job for what it was, an honest living with good pay, good benefits and a pension after twenty years. Tens of thousands of people take the test for Sanitation every four years and only a small percentage get the call to join. When I was at my worst, I used to beg God for a regular life. Now, with over a year of sobriety behind me, and the opportunity at a solid career for the city I lived in, I had everything I needed to live that life I once prayed for. I went to the appointment, retook a few medical tests, and got my hire date. At 0600 hours on August 21, 2006 at Floyd Bennett Field in Brooklyn, New York, I would start my career and officially become one of New York's Strongest.

Training was two weeks. At first it was a lot of speeches from higher ups in the department and union delegates followed by an enormous amount of paperwork. I was so excited I didn't care how boring the topic was, I was all ears, all day. When all the paperwork was out of the way, we took to the field. We drove department equipment through various obstacle courses set up by the training staff.. We learned how to dump a truck, change a tire, properly lift a garbage can and attach a plow to a big orange salt spreader. We did two nights of training in the field doing relays, which is driving trucks to the dump, emptying them and returning them to the garage for the next shift. Patty had been an instructor at Floyd Bennet the last two years. Having him there made it a lot easier. Because I was his friend, the other instructors looked out for me and gave me more detailed training, plus, I didn't have a car yet, so he picked me up every morning. Patty was always good to me. He always reached out even when nobody else would, and I made a mess of it every time. There was a time in our lives when we were inseparable. I missed not having that bond anymore so those two weeks of riding in together every morning brought back a lot of good memories. Training was coming to an end to an end and we were about to get our assignments. There was a guy in the meetings who had a friend in the union and he swore up and down for a year that he would get me anywhere I wanted to go when I got hired. When push finally came to shove, he couldn't get me in any of the spots I wanted, but he was able to keep me in Brooklyn. I had a choice of three spots, and with his advice, I chose a small garage in Crown Heights. I was the only guy assigned there and when the instructors at Floyd Bennett heard where I was going, they all made the sign of the cross. I immediately regretted my decision, having a fear of the unknown world I was about to enter, but that fear would be unwarranted. On September 11, 2006 I would start my career at BK9. The small garage in Crown Heights, and the men and women who worked there would become a staple in my life for years to come.

CHAPTER 26

Life is Good.

I heard from many people over the years say that the Department of Sanitation was the best job in the city and the equivalent of hitting the lotto. Let's be honest, if I hit the lotto I wouldn't be working for any department, anywhere, but I understood the meaning behind the words. I knew I was lucky. I was lucky that my mother forced me to take the test three years earlier. I was lucky that my list number was called. Most of all I was lucky to be alive to answer the call when it came. The timing couldn't have been better. If the call came in 2004, I would've lasted three days before my alcohol and drug use got me canned. If it came in 2005, I may have never built the foundation I did in recovery or had the experience working for Imperial, which gave me a whole new outlook on putting in an honest days work. I was grateful for the opportunity I was blessed with and I was proud to put on the uniform. From day one I was willing to do any task assigned to me to the best of my ability.

My first day on the job I got there extra early. Everyone I met welcomed me warmly, the Superintendent introduced himself and told me a little bit about the way things work. I signed in, sat on a chair leaning on the wall by the diesel gas pump, and waited for my assignment to come. When six o'clock came, the volume increased. Dozens of guys and two women crowded the garage floor and listened for their name to be read off the roll call sheet. Cards were given out with assignments, and crew after crew grabbed their stuff and went to their trucks. When the noise settled down, the Supervisor called my name. I walked to the yellow guardrail that separated the front office from the garage floor.

"Figlioli, you're with Makluski. You guys are on MLP. He knows what to do. Be careful out there. Have a good day."

MLP is Motorized Litter Patrol. You're given a route, a garbage pail, a broom and a shovel. You go out and you sweep the streets. Simple as that. If you were lucky enough to get a truck, the afternoon would usually consist of emptying a few avenues of corner baskets or drop offs. Drop offs are bulk garbage "dropped off" at various locations by unknown perpetrators. They are usually called in to the city's 311 complaint system who directs them to the responsible city agency. Getting drop-offs or baskets was a good thing, because you got to be in the truck most of the afternoon and it made the day go a little quicker. Makluski was a good guy, he was on the job a little over a year and gave me the rundown of the whole district. He told me who the good guys were and who to stay away from. He gave me tips on everything from how to drive the truck to the best places to eat in the neighborhood. We were assigned Utica Avenue from Eastern Parkway to Empire Boulevard. That area at that time of day is insane. There's a subway station and ten different busses. You have illegal taxis picking up and dropping off people by the dozens all morning long. The amount of people is mind-blowing. The amount of litter is ridiculous. You sweep a block and ten minutes later its filthy again. It really is a losing battle, but I loved every minute of it. From where my life was two years earlier to where it was now, I couldn't be more grateful, and that was a good thing, because I would spend the next year of my life sweeping Utica Avenue by day and picking up corner baskets on the overnight shift. It was a grind, and my sleep schedule was all messed up, but like anything in life, you must pay your dues. I was happily paying them daily and making friend after friend along the way. It would take another book to fit them all but, George, Jimmy, Guy, Ralph, Mike, John, Vinny, Anthony, Danny, Mike, Denis, Rudy, Howie, Julio and Steve are just some of the names of BK9 that I would work with over the years and come to call my friend.

It was the summer of 2007 and things were about as good as they ever were. I was going on two and a half years sober and I was about to pass my probationary period with the Department. I would always say that all I needed was a good job and a good girl to get my life together. It turns out I needed to get my life together first for those things to come. Everything was falling into place, but there was still something missing. I was lonely. It had been almost five years since I felt anything serious for anyone. There were random girls here and there, but nothing of any substance and none since I became sober. They say you shouldn't date anyone in your first year and I took that seriously. In my second year I went on two dates. The first was with a woman who was ten years older than me that I met in a tattoo shop. She was what we in recovery refer to as a civilian, or someone who has never been a part of our world. Over dinner I proceeded to tell her about some of my less than stellar moments over the years. It turns out no civilian woman wants to hear about bookmaking, crack smoking and psych wards on the first date. The second date was with a girl I met at a meeting. The stories told at that dinner were enough to put us both in jail for a long time, and while there's something oddly hot about a girl pistol whipping somebody that sold her bad drugs, I didn't think she was the one for me. Now, five months into year three, with no real prospects, I was starting to think it just wasn't in the cards for me to meet the right girl. That's when she walked into my life. It was a Thursday night at the Fresh and by now, me and Stevie Mags pretty much had every commitment in the place. We would open the doors every week, set up the chairs, make the coffee, count the money and clean up when the meeting ended. We did it all. When seven thirty rolled around, she came through the door and sat about ten chairs away from me. She was beautiful. She had dark hair, dark eyes and was well built with a perfect tan. A week earlier someone asked me what kind of girl I was attracted to and my answer described her. The meeting started and we went around the room. When it got to her, she introduced herself and said a few words. I liked what she said and I liked how she said it. She was sober around five years and she seemed to have her life together. I liked the way she walked, and I liked the way she laughed. Without knowing this girl at all, I liked everything about her. I liked her so much that I did nothing. She was intimidating and my fear of rejection overtook me. I let her walk out the door that night without saying a word.

When I woke up Friday morning, the thought of the night before haunted me. How did I let that girl walk out without saying anything? Here I am thirty-one years old, still afraid to talk to a pretty girl. I was in a bad mood all day. A few guys at work asked me what was wrong and I said nothing. They would torture my life if I told them I saw girl I liked last night, but I didn't talk to her because I was afraid. When I got off work I called Stevie. I laid it all out there for him, my feelings, my fear, everything. When I was done ranting he didn't even try to be serious, he once again told me to eat a chocolate bar. I couldn't help but laugh. It had to sound crazy. Here I was, a grown man telling another grown man that I was afraid to talk to a girl. It wasn't crazy though. I was afraid to talk to pretty girls when I was fifteen and I solved that by drinking alcohol. When I drank, the fear went away. That's how I dealt with my whole life. Now I was thirty-one and sober, but that fear never left because I never learned how to do things any other way. The woman in the tattoo shop talked to me first. When we went on the date, I was so nervous and lost for words that I said things I shouldn't have. The other girl was a progression. We knew each other from a group setting. Small talk built up over six months so it was easy to ask her out. Once we were out, we had so much in common, there were no nerves. This was different because I would have to initiate a conversation with someone I didn't know, someone I was intimidated by, without the help of any substances. I had to be myself, and I didn't know how to do that. That was the great thing about the meetings. You could go to people with problems like these and you weren't judged. You could always find someone who went through the same thing and get guidance on how to get through it. Stevie gave me no such guidance, but he did offer a solution. His girlfriend at the time happened to know the girl from the meeting. She was willing to put a good word in for me, but I would have to make the first move once she did. That sounded like a good plan to me. I would spend the next six days preparing myself for my big moment. What would I say to her if I got the green light? I played it out a million times in my head. I was an absolute nervous wreck. Thursday night came and I was bursting with anticipation. I had the words rehearsed in my head. I would be funny and I would be charming. All I needed was the green light. They say when you make plans, God laughs. He was rolling on the floor that night because she didn't show up to the meeting. Stevie's girlfriend did give me some good news. She talked to the girl from the meeting, and I had the green light to do my thing. The nerves settled down and I felt good about the situation. I had another week to tighten up my opening line and another week of not facing my fear. Once again God was laughing. I got to the Fresh late the following night and the meeting had already started. When I walked in there she was, sitting directly next to the door. We couldn't help but come face to face, but the meeting was in progress, so we just exchanged a smile. I took my seat next to Stevie, who tortured me the entire meeting about following through with my part in the master plan. The meeting ended and I helped clean up as usual. I was moving slower than normal and Stevie noticed.

"She's going to leave kid, you better go talk to her or someone else will scoop her up." He said sarcastically.

I finally finished up and climbed the stairs. I felt like I was walking to the electric chair. Talking to a girl shouldn't be this hard. Worst case scenario she turns me away. That's not a big deal for most, but in my head it was. I cared what other people thought about me so much, that any chink in the armor of the reputation I built for myself in the Fresh, would be devastating. Truth was that these people liked me for me, and nobody really cared that much about my dating life to give it a second thought one way or another. I slowly walked over to her, rehearsing the words in my head. It felt like an eternity to walk the ten-foot distance between us. I came up behind her, tapped her on the shoulder and the words I had been putting together in my head for the last seven days were nowhere to be found. My insides started to shake, my underarms started to sweat, and in that moment I went back to the most basic form of introduction I knew. I put out my hand and said,

"Hi, I'm Tommy."

She looked at me and flashed a pretty, yet bashful smile. She was just as nervous as I was. She shook my hand firmly and said,

"Hi, I'm Julie."

There was a moment of silence, so I pulled out a cigarette and asked for a light. She lit my cigarette and that broke the ice. She asked me where I lived and what I did for a living. When I told her I was on Sanitation she asked if I knew her Cousin Mike. Earlier that day I was working out of town at another district in the zone. When she told me his last name, I realized that I worked with him that morning. Over six thousand sanitation workers and this girls cousin is the one I worked with hours before introducing myself to her. I saw that as a sign from God and my nerves instantly disappeared. We were so focused on each other that by the time we ended our conversation everybody had left. We exchanged phone numbers and made plans to see each other the following week. She kissed me on the cheek, flashed her pretty smile, got in her car and drove away. I felt like a million dollars, all the fear and anxiety was gone. All the time I spent trying to come up with what I thought she wanted to hear was for nothing. In the end all I had to do was be myself.

CHAPTER 27

Snap, Crackle, Pop, It's Only One.

As 2008 rolled around, life was as good as it ever was. By now me and Julie had been together five months and the job was going great. I passed my probation and my garage was assigned ten new guys out of class to replenish our numbers. With ten guys below me in seniority, my work schedule became a bit steadier and it gave me more time for my personal life. Growing up I always looked forward to Christmas Eve dinner at my house. Aunt Eileen would host, and it was the one night a year that the whole family would get together. To present day, Christmas Eve is still my favorite night of the year. Julie's family had that type of get together every week. Sunday dinner at her Uncle Carl's house was a tradition that I quickly came to look forward to. Carl and his family were honest, blue collar, hardworking people. It didn't take long for me to admire him, his wife, and the life they made for themselves and their children. I would find myself driving and being overcome with moments of absolute gratitude and serenity. My life was in shambles three years earlier, now, I had a great job, a beautiful girlfriend, and for the first time in my life I was looking up to the right kind of people. The people in the meetings told me if I just kept coming around and doing the right thing, my life would get better. I followed those instructions and the life I was promised was revealing itself more and more with each passing day.

It was a week before my three-year anniversary. It was my last day at work before my vacation started and I was on one of the better recycling routes in the district. On this day I was working with J. Pratt, who can only be described as an acquired taste. He was a great guy once you got to know him, but he was very loud and set in his ways. Guys didn't want to work with him for that reason and he would always wind up with the most junior guy on the shift. Early in my career I didn't love working with him, but I had no choice, so I would suck it up and make the best of it. As we were nearing the end of the route, I pulled up to a big bag stop. Stops like these need two people to load, so I popped the parking brake, grabbed my gloves and stepped out of the truck. For some reason I didn't look down before I exited the vehicle, and I stepped directly into a pothole with all my body weight landing on my left leg. As soon as my foot hit the hole, my ankle turned over and a sharp pain shot up my entire body. I fell to the floor and yelled in agony. Pratt ran around the truck and saw me laying on the ground. Without hesitation he scooped me up in a fireman carry and put me back in the truck. He got on his phone and called the supervisor to come transport me to the hospital. My ankle was throbbing and I was afraid to look at the damage I had done. He spent the next fifteen minutes telling me everything would be good, that injuries were part of the job. When the supervisor arrived at the scene, Pratt threw me over his shoulder yet again and carried me to the car. He told me to feel better and finished the route by himself. From that day on I had a new respect for Pratt. His actions that day showed me the good person he was underneath all the bravado and working with him became something I enjoyed doing.

I was transported to Kings County Hospital, which is one of the top trauma hospitals in the city. If you're shot, stabbed or sustained any other life threatening injuries, this is the place to go. For a possible broken ankle, not so much. You would think being in uniform would get me some preferential treatment, but it did not. I spent the next eight hours sitting in a wheelchair in the waiting room. It wasn't until I made a grievance with the patient service coordinator that I was seen. Apparently their computers were down, so my triage records never made it through the system. They never knew I was even there. I was finally seen by a doctor and after x-rays came back negative, I was wrapped up, given a set of crutches and told to follow up with an orthopedic doctor. This was my first experience with a LODI or line of duty injury. The process is a pain in the ass, and being it was my first time, I was like a deer in headlights when I reported to the department medical facility the next morning. Long story short, I was given authorization to see an orthopedic specialist and told to report back two weeks later. It turned out to be a grade two sprain with partially torn ligaments. My ankle looked like a softball and was three different shades of purple. I was in a good deal of pain, but when I was offered Vicodin, I didn't even consider accepting them. I told the doctor I was an addict and that I couldn't take narcotic medication. He told me he admired my honesty and gave me Ibuprofen 800 to help with the pain. March 12th came and I celebrated my third anniversary on crutches, in a snowstorm. The crowd was lighter than the previous two years because of the weather, but all the important people were there. Dougie and Betty spoke for me, and my family and friends showed up along with Julie and her mom. When I accepted my coin, I was able to reflect on how much my life had changed over the last three years. I brought up the incident of turning down the painkillers which was met by a big round of applause. You can talk about it in meetings and play it out in your head a million times. Until you're presented with the situation, you never know how you will react. I was proud of how I handled it and I was proud of the change I made. One more milestone was in the books and the words Dougie said to me after my first anniversary came to mind. What comes after three years? I went home, took some Ibuprofen, put my leg up and thought to myself, three years and a day kid, three years and a day.

I spent the next six weeks rehabbing my ankle and returned to work in the middle of May. I had been seeing Julie for ten months now, and the honeymoon period had just about run its course. We would argue over small insignificant things and often say things that were hurtful to each other. The thing with this situation was that this was the first real relationship either one of us had been in sober. You can't just walkout and get high or drink the feelings away, you had to deal with them head on. That's where meetings and guys like Dougie and Stevie came in. When I was dealing with anything new, I would run it across them, and they would try to steer me in the right direction according to their life experiences. For some reason I wasn't forthcoming with the disagreements me and Julie were having, and I chose to process all the feelings on my own. We would fight and make up a few times a month and I would just chalk it up to normal couples bullshit. It was during this time that Julie became increasingly negative towards the meetings and started frequenting another recovery program for issues she had not relating to alcohol and drugs. I too started to scale back on the number of meetings I attended choosing to spend most of my free time with her. It was the summer of 2008 and it got to the point that I was only attending meetings at the Fresh two nights a week. When I did go, I would get there early and eat dinner with Stevie, Dougie, and some of the new members I had become friends with. When the meeting started, I would hang out in the kitchen and not pay attention to what was being said by the speaker. I started to become judgmental of things people shared and I would find myself complaining about it to Julie when we were together. Instead of changing things up and going to different meetings, I chose to scale back even more, going only once a week and resenting every second I was there. When people would ask why I wasn't around as much, I would just say I was busy with work, or that me and Julie had plans. It was a dangerous game I was playing, but at no point did I think my sobriety was in any danger. I figured it to be a phase, and after a while I would find the passion again for the program that helped me turn my life around.

The summer was moving along, and as the calendar changed to August I was about to complete my second year with Sanitation. Me and Julie's first anniversary together was approaching and the arguing that had dominated most of the spring and early summer had subsided. I was grateful for my relationship and grateful for my job. As cynical as my attitude had been of late, I was looking forward to celebrating these milestones in my life. One morning while on a collection route, I bent down to pick up a bag and I felt a slight pull in my lower back. When I straightened up to put the bag in the truck the pull turned to a pain. When I tried to take a step, the pain increased. I rested for a few minutes, but that just made it worse. It tightened up and I could barely move at all. Here we go again, just three months after returning from my ankle injury, I would once again have to go out on medical leave for a line of duty injury. The process at Kings County was better this time around. The nurse who triaged me had family on the job so she fast tracked me through the system. When all was said and done, I only spent a few hours in the hospital. When the x-rays showed nothing out of the ordinary, I was given Ibuprofen for pain, and instructions to follow up with an orthopedic doctor as soon as possible. I went down to the department health facility and it wasn't nearly as intimidating this time around. I knew what to expect and I found that if you approach most of the doctors there with a modicum of respect, they usually treated you the right way. I got my authorization to see the orthopedic and my orders to report back in two weeks. As I was leaving, I ran into a guy from my garage. He had been out with a back injury for months and we started to catch up. I didn't love the doctor I went to for my ankle. I felt the rehab process was severely lacking and it caused my recovery time to go on longer than it should have. I asked who he used, and he gave me the card to his doctor in Bay Ridge, having nothing but good things to say about him. As we parted ways, knowing my past issues from conversations we had over the last two years, he looked at me and said,

"Just be careful. He's a little free with his prescription pad."

I chuckled, thanked him for the recommendation, then went home and made an appointment to see the doctor the following week.

On the day of the appointment I got to the office a half hour early. I filled out the necessary paperwork and they took me down to the lab for further x-rays on my back. I went back to the waiting room and after twenty minutes I was called into the office. When the doctor walked in, he was exactly how my friend described. He was soft spoken and thorough. He spoke all the important details of the exam into a small recording device he kept in his coat pocket. His initial assessment was a pulled muscle that should get better in a few weeks with the proper rest, but he suggested I get an MRI to rule out any herniation of my discs. I've seen what back problems do to people and at thirty-two years old that was the last thing I wanted. His diagnosis and the test to rule out any major damage was exactly what I wanted to hear. Just when I thought the appointment couldn't have gone any better, he asked me one last question. He asked me if I was in pain. The words of my friend telling me how the doctor was free with his prescription pad popped into my head. I knew what his response would be if I answered yes. I went back and forth in my head for a moment and said that I was in a bit of pain. It wasn't a lie. I was in pain, but that pain was perfectly controlled with the Ibuprofen the hospital gave me. He took his pad out, wrote me a script and handed it to me. I slowly brought it into focus, and it read, Vicodin 7.5/750/#40/1tab/t.i.d/as needed for pain, refill four times. I looked at the words and my mind went quiet. I felt like I was the only person in the room. I knew the words written on that paper well. I had written them myself just four years earlier. My stomach tightened and my blood filled with adrenaline. There was that old familiar feeling from way back when. I knew what I needed to do. I had to tell him the truth, that I was an addict and I couldn't take the script. I did it just a few months earlier when I hurt my ankle and was offered the same. This time I didn't. I got up and left the office with the script in my pocket and drove to the Rite Aid just ten blocks from my house. I sat in the car for a half hour going back and forth in my head about what to do. There was only one answer, but my mind wouldn't accept it. I made one wrong choice by accepting the script in the first place, but there was still time to make it right. I had to call someone and tell them what was going on. Even though I had been detached from meetings lately, I still knew what to do. I picked up my phone and dialed my friend Chris. Chris, or Little Chris as we called him, came into my life around the same time as Julie. We were the same age and had a lot of the same interests. We had grown to be good friends over the last year and with a history of opiate use in his story, I knew he was the one who would understand what I was going through most. He picked up the phone and talked to me for an hour. I told him I was struggling with the decision and he simply ended the conversation with, throw the script in the garbage and come to my house. I hung the phone up, got out of my car and as if I were on autopilot, I walked into Rite Aid and I filled the prescription. I didn't stand a chance. The truth was that I made the decision a week earlier when my friend warned me about the doctor. I knew he would offer me painkillers and deep down I think I wanted them. I drove to Chris's house and left the pills in my car. I went up to his apartment, ate dinner, played video games and thanked him for talking me out of a bad decision. I went home, put the pills in my dresser drawer, and went to sleep.

For the next two weeks I woke up every morning and went downstairs to eat cereal and drink a Manhattan Special. Every morning I would have the pills in my pocket and I would wrestle with the idea of taking one. I didn't call anyone and I didn't pray. Everything I learned in my three years and five months of sobriety was being dominated by the thoughts of taking only one. It had been so long and my back was killing me. What's one pill going to do? I told myself those lies repeatedly until one morning I couldn't hold it back any longer. I opened the bottle and took out one pill. I put it in my mouth and the bitter taste brought me right back to 2004. I grabbed the Manhattan Special and I washed it down. I finished the rest of my cereal and I watched tv for another half hour. For a moment I thought I got away with it. The minimal pain in my back was gone and I didn't feel high. Maybe I would be ok. Maybe this wouldn't be such a bad thing. I got up to bring my bowl to the kitchen and that's when it hit me, the sense of warmth and well-being only an opiate can bring. I was so detached from my recovery that the pill I took that day was just the physical relapse. Mentally I had already been checked out for months. It was in that moment I realized the enormity of the decision I made, but it was too late. The beast was awake and now I would have to deal with all that would come with it.

CHAPTER 28

Living A Lie

After the first Vicodin, I found myself staring at my watch, patiently waiting for six hours to pass so I could take another. I kept telling myself to take only one, figuring if I followed the instructions on the bottle it wasn't a relapse. When the time came, I did take one, but I followed it with five Manhattan Specials, figuring the extra jolt of caffeine would speed up the euphoric effect. It's things like that you don't realize in the moment, but looking back, you realize how crazy it was. This routine would go on for a few more days. I would take one every six hours, only now my back wasn't hurting anymore. I still tried to justify it to myself, but it was apparent this had nothing to do with pain and everything to do with chasing a feeling. A few more days would pass, and I started to grow a tolerance to one every six hours, so I started taking two. I quickly realized where this was going, so I called Julie and asked her to come get the pills and bring them to her house. I told her I didn't trust myself and it was better if she held them and gave them to me if needed. I hadn't built a physical dependency yet so there was no sickness when I stopped taking them, but the mental obsession was there, and it was as strong as it ever had been. A few months passed and I was back to work. I wound up flushing the rest of the pills knowing that I would've finished the bottle otherwise. I knew my intentions behind taking them, and deep down I knew it was a relapse, but the more time that passed, the easier it was to justify what I did and forget it ever happened. I started going back to meetings, but I never said a word about it. As the year turned to 2009, the Vicodin incident started to become a distant afterthought.

March rolled around and I celebrated my four-year anniversary at the Fresh. When I was handed my four-year coin, I couldn't even look at it, knowing it wasn't real, the guilt ate at my soul. People would ask me to speak at meetings and I would refuse, guys would ask me to sponsor them and I would say no. Everything I took pride in doing wasn't an option anymore because I knew I was a fraud. I needed something to stop the feelings of guilt and shame, to fill the hole the relapse created. I didn't want to get high, but I couldn't come clean. Instead, I decided to buy an engagement ring for Julie, and I asked her to marry me shortly after my fraudulent anniversary. I proposed at Mohegan Sun at her father's award ceremony. Her father was a renowned foot doctor and that's all I really have to say about him. They weren't close and I was glad because he wasn't a nice guy. I asked his blessing out of respect, but I didn't care one way or another what he said. Her mom and Uncle were on board and that's all the blessing I needed. The one thing I will give him credit for is that he knew it wasn't a good idea. I didn't see it at the time, but I believe he was looking out for my well-being more than I was. He knew his daughter, and he knew she was tough to deal with. He asked me if I was sure about what I was doing and I said yes. When I want to do something, I do it, regardless of what anyone thinks about it, once the thought is stuck in my head, consider it a done deal. I had a whole plan concocted in my head, but halfway through the night, he said something that upset her, and she wound up in the room crying for hours. With no way of getting her to the area I originally planned, I asked her in the room. She said yes and the tears disappeared. We told everybody the news and the rest of the weekend was a good time. We got home and spent the next week going around to all our friends showing off the ring and our happiness. We started to make plans in our heads, nothing real, just fantasy options of our future wedding. Three months later we had a party at a restaurant in my neighborhood where our friends and family gathered to celebrate our engagement. After the party we sat in her house and opened our gifts. People were very generous, and we made out like bandits. We were set to move into a new apartment at the beginning of July and all appeared great on the outside, but inside I was struggling. The excitement of the engagement made me forget about the relapse. When it was all over, the guilt came back. It was all fake. I could paint a pretty picture to show everyone else, but facts remained that I was living a lie. I wasn't the person they all thought I was. These feelings were relentless, and I couldn't shake them. The next day we were leaving to spend a few days in Atlantic City with her mom, aunt, and Uncle Carl. I got up early that morning, telling her I needed to pick something up from my house before we left. I drove home and went into my dresser drawer. I took the empty bottle of Vicodin that I had flushed months earlier and read the side of the bottle. I dialed the pharmacy number and requested my first of four refills. I picked them up, opened the bottle, and without hesitation washed four pills down with a sugar free red bull. I never came clean and I never dealt with the feelings that were the cause and effect of the my actions in the first place. The relapse never ended, it just lay dormant. There was no more fooling myself and no more trying to take just one. I wanted the feelings to go away and instead of facing them head on I chose the only other route I knew. I chose to get high.

CHAPTER 29

Coming Clean

I moved into my new place on Bay 11th Street in Bath Beach, Brooklyn on July 1st. It was a ground floor, split level, one bedroom, with a small kitchen, small living room, and two bathrooms. It was perfect for a couples first apartment together and I was looking forward to my new living arrangement. The only problem was that Julie decided she didn't want to leave her mother's house, and she waited until that day to break the news. This hurt me on two different levels. The first being the obvious disappointment of Julie wanting to live with her mother instead of me. The second was that I budgeted everything on two people living there. I wasn't at top pay yet with the department, so all my expenses doubling with her last minute decision left me in a bad financial spot from day one. My daily Vicodin intake was steadily increasing, and the stress of my new financial burden just furthered my use of the drug. I was able to get four more refills from my orthopedic by telling him my back still bothered me on a daily basis, but knowing that well would dry up sooner or later I had to start looking for another source. Brinsley always said I could find a drug dealer in a sea of saints. This time I didn't have to find him, he found me.

It was my first night at the apartment and I was sitting outside smoking a cigarette with my landlord Rick. A guy walked up to where we were sitting, shook hands with Rick and engaged in some small talk. When they were finished, I was introduced to the new face. His name was Marco and he lived in the upstairs apartment with his parents. Rick excused himself to go inside for the night and me and Marco started talking. As soon as he opened his mouth, I knew exactly what he was. I feel like drug dealers and users alike have a sense for each other. He must've had that sense for me just as I had for him. Within twenty minutes of speaking, he told me the bar he spent most of his time in and the people he associated with. He gave me the rundown of what he can get, the amount he could get, and the price he could get it for. It took less than eight hours in my new surroundings to find what I wanted. Within three months I was taking between thirty and forty Vicodin or Percocet a day. I would wake up in the morning and take just enough to straighten out. I would take enough during the day to keep a slight buzz, then when I got home, I would take them by the handfuls until I passed out wherever I happened to be sitting. Many an early morning I would be woken up by my alarm, nodded out on the toilet bowl or passed out on the bathroom floor. On top of me having trouble making ends meet with my bills, I now had a two hundred dollar a day pill habit on top of it. It started to show in my appearance and one night my mother commented on how bad my skin looked. I told her I wasn't sleeping right and working on the truck was taking a toll on me. She accepted my excuses, but she knew something was wrong, as she always said, a mother knows. To combat this, I just stopped going to see her. I stopped going to meetings completely because a room full of people like me would know as soon as they saw me what was going on. Stevie and Little Chris would reach out often, but after a while they stopped, realizing there was not much they could do to reign me back in, they left it in the hands of God. By now Dougie had been diagnosed with stage four lung cancer and in his final days he was struggling with opiates just as I was. Seeing him like that hurt me deeply, and instead of being the man and friend I should've been, I stopped going to see him as well. I spent all my spare time getting high and hanging out at Julie's house. She wasn't getting high with me and I don't think she knew what was going on, but it was taking its toll on both of us. My moods swung violently and it didn't take much to send me into a state of misery. I was unhappy in the relationship and still pissed off about her hanging me out to dry on the apartment. I would start fights over everything, often storming out of her house to go home and be with who I really wanted to be with, my pills, and myself.

Work was getting to be an issue as well. I was calling out sick often, and when I was there I wasn't myself. I was stressed out all the time, worrying about being drug tested. At the time, the federal DOT drug test wasn't looking for synthetic opiates, but I didn't know that. I would wait until five minutes before roll call every day to sign in, then avoid driving the truck as much as possible during the day. I would be ok in the morning until the euphoria from my first dose wore off, then my mood would turn sour. I found myself snapping at guys in the garage for no reason, and it was often the people I was closest to. As 2009 came to an end, my life was once again spinning out of control and I needed something to snap it back in the right direction.

It was February 7, 2010. It was Super Bowl Sunday, but the last thing on my mind that day was football. I was struggling greatly and it became harder to hold it together with each passing day. They say God puts people in your life when you need them the most. On this day it wasn't a person, but a dog, that would help me see the light. I stayed at Julie's the night before and woke up on the couch, groggy and in withdrawal, as was the norm with the level my pill consumption had gotten to. I grabbed a handful of Vicodin and drank a cup of coffee. As I sat in the living room Julie's dog Jackson came running over to me. Jackson was a gigantic golden retriever with an equally gigantic personality. He was by far, the craziest dog I ever met in my life. He wouldn't listen to anybody and he ate everything from food to umbrellas. One night I made the mistake of leaving a new dress shirt I bought at Kohls on the kitchen table. I went upstairs for twenty minutes and when I came down he had eaten part of the collar. I had to bring it back to Kohls and explain the situation to the customer service person. They got such a kick out of it, they not only replaced the shirt, but gave me another one for free in case it happened again. Despite his crazy ways, I loved that dog. I would take him for walks whenever I was there, and at over one hundred pounds, he would attempt to sit on my lap any chance he got. We developed such a bond that there were times I would go there just to see him and leave before Julie got home. That morning he started with his usual attempt to get on my lap, followed by his attempt to eat my sneaker. Once he calmed down he just sat there in front of me. As I was petting him, I found myself telling him everything I was going through. All the things I wouldn't tell anyone else I told Jackson. I told him of the relapse, my struggles financially, my mood swings, my guilt, my shame, and my sadness. I put my head down and broke out in tears. Jackson, in the most gentle way he knew how, put his paws on my shoulders, put his head next to mine, and started crying with me. Jackson took my sadness as his own and he consoled me. He showed me it was ok to come clean about everything, that I wouldn't be ridiculed or judged, I would be understood and taken care of. I left the house and called Little Chris, I told him I relapsed and it had gotten out of control. He told me he had been waiting on my call since he figured it out for himself many months earlier. He told me he would help me. That night he came to my apartment with his girlfriend Marissa to watch the Super Bowl and talk about our plan going forward. A weight was lifted from my shoulders that day, and I felt that everything would be ok. All I needed to do was be honest and ask for help.

CHAPTER 30

Welcome to the Darkside!

Despite Chris advising against it, I decided my best path to getting clean again was to go on a Suboxone program. I didn't want too many people finding out about my relapse, and with my financial situation being where it was, I didn't want to miss out on the overtime coming my way with a big snowstorm quickly approaching. I saw the doctor Tuesday morning and we went over my options. He asked me about my history with opiate use and questioned why I never went back to Oxycontin. My simple answer was that I couldn't find them and if I did this would be a very different conversation. When all was said and done, he outlined his plan for me. I would start on sixteen milligrams a day and titrate down over eighteen months until I was off the drug and fully reestablished in my recovery. He wrote me the first prescription and I waited outside the pharmacy for it to be filled. I was already in withdrawal, which is a prerequisite for the first dose of Suboxone, so the wait was slightly uncomfortable to say the least. Once filled, I took my first dose and reported back to the doctor. It worked wonders. The withdrawal went away and I didn't feel high. With the help of Suboxone and support from my twelve-step community, I was confident that I could get myself back on the right track.

My relationship with Julie was all but dead. We spent most of 2010 breaking up and getting back together. There was no love anymore, it was about comfort and codependency. Everyone around us saw how toxic it had become, but neither one of us were ready to let go completely. The first breakup occurred shortly after I started going back to meetings. To take my mind off things I joined a local gym. I figured between work, meetings and the gym, I wouldn't have time to think about where the relationship went wrong. Shortly after starting the gym I befriended a neighborhood guy named Donny. Donny was one of the nicest people I ever came across. He lived a few blocks away from me with his mom and Donny loved to talk. The guy talked nonstop. If he was spotting me on a bench-press, he would physically follow the bar up and down in order to not skip a beat in whatever conversation we were having. Donny, much like me, struggled with addiction his whole life, and like me, was trying to get his life back together. There was an instant bond between us, and we would wind up spending a lot of time together over the next few years. I also ran into a face from the past. His name was Sally Boy. He was one of the older kids from the block I grew up on and out of them all, he was the one I looked up to the most. His dad, a flashy street guy who reminded me a lot of my own father, was murdered in 1985 and after that Sally Boy was never the same. He spent most of his life in and out of trouble, participating in one scheme after the next. Also, like myself, he struggled with addiction most of his adult life. As crazy as it sounds, his faults were a big part of the reason I looked up to him. He worked down the block from the gym at an insurance company owned by a neighborhood guy. It had been about fifteen years since I last saw him , but not much changed. At thirty-four and thirty-nine years old, he still referred to me as Little Figgy and I still looked up to him like I was a little kid. I had been eating right and working out for a few months by now, and it was starting to show. I felt great and looked great as well. As we were saying our goodbyes, he looked me up and down and said,

"Figgy, you look good, but we gotta start sticking some needles in you and get you some size."

I laughed it off and commented back that steroids weren't my thing. He chuckled as well, and we exchanged numbers, planning to keep in touch and work out together a few days a week. As I continued my workout after he left, his words echoed in my head. I gazed around the gym, noticing everybody's seemingly overnight gains and my mind started to work overtime. The Jersey Shore television show was in its infancy stages and girls loved those guys, girls loved Sally Boy as well. I thought to myself, *I'm no different than these guys, all I need is the muscles.* Much like associating cigarettes and alcohol with being able to talk to girls I was otherwise afraid to approach twenty years earlier, I associated it now with looking a certain way. I was about to start my life again post Julie and the insecurity and fear of doing so took over my entire being. That night, at Sally Boys apartment in Staten Island, he filled a syringe with a yellow tinted, oily liquid and stuck it in my left shoulder. The substance was Testosterone Cypionate. Sure, I wasn't getting high on opiates or drinking my feelings away, but my lifetime insecurities and belief that I wasn't good enough never went away. You can put down drugs and alcohol, but until you deal with the underlying issues, those feelings never go away. You will spend your entire life trying to suppress them with whatever you could find. As a child I did it by doing things other people told me to do in order for them to like me. As I got older, I did it with cigarettes, gambling, alcohol, drugs and people. I tried to portray myself as someone I wasn't as far back as I could remember, and this was no different. I wasn't comfortable in my own skin and I wasn't willing to wait the time it would take to look the way I wanted. That night I found my answer, and that night would start my journey into the use of anabolic steroids. As he withdrew the needle from my shoulder, he looked at me with a grin and said,

" Welcome to the Darkside pal!"

CHAPTER 31

Diana

I started injecting 400mg's of Test Cyp every week. Two hundred on Tuesday and two hundred on Thursday was my weekly routine. I quickly got used to giving myself the shots and in a little over a month I had put on twenty pounds, most of it in muscle. I looked better than ever and I felt just as good. By Memorial Day of 2010, people started to notice my transformation, which I attributed to eating a lot more and working my ass off every day at the gym. Don't get me wrong, both were true. You can't just stick a needle in your ass twice a week, sit on the couch eating ring dings, and expect to see results. I was breaking my ass every day, but the steroids were the reason it was all happening so quickly. People accepted my explanation as truth, but I'm sure there were many who knew what I was up to. I guess they figured as long as I wasn't getting high on painkillers, a little testosterone wasn't going to kill me. Me and Julie met for coffee one night and decided to give it another shot. In lasted less than a month and it was over yet again. Donny, Sally Boy, Little Chris, guys at work and even her own family would yell at me all the time, telling me the relationship wasn't worth the stress it was putting in my life. As July rolled around, I decided it was time to move on. I made a profile on a few dating sites and put some feelers out around the meetings and neighborhood. I talked to a few girls through the sites and one or two at the gym. I went on a few dates with one of them, but there wasn't any spark to speak of. One day I got a message on my phone. I can't remember the exact words, but it was something like *hello Brooklyn boy*. I went on my computer and it was from the website HotorNot.com. Hot or Not was a site that you put a picture on for people to rate from one through ten. Me and a guy from the gym made a bet one day on who would get a better rating. We both took the most obnoxious pictures possible in front of the mirror in the gyms basement and uploaded them to the site. Someone saw my picture and sent me a message. When I went on the site and saw the girl who sent it, I thought it was a robot. She was beautiful. She had dark hair, a killer smile and the tiny dress she was wearing in the picture made her ass look fantastic. I figured I'd give it a shot, so I messaged her back, *hello Staten Island girl.* A few hours later I got a response and we wound up talking back and forth the rest of the night. Neither one of us had a paid subscription to the site, so I guess there were forces greater than ourselves at work that day. Whatever the case was, we exchanged phone numbers and texted back and forth for the next few days. One night she called me, and we spent two hours on the phone, talking about everything from what we liked to eat to what kind of tanning method we liked the most. Her name was Diana. She lived on the South Shore of Staten Island with her parents and two brothers. She was a lot younger than me, about to turn twenty-two, but there was something about the way she spoke that made her seem mature beyond her years. I had to meet this girl. She was going on vacation with a friend for two weeks, so we made plans to meet each other when she returned.

As the two weeks passed, I went back and forth in my head about whether this was the right thing to do. The age difference was the biggest problem I was having. When I confided in a few friends at work they assured me that if I didn't meet her, one of them would gladly take my place. The day came that we were going to meet and up until the last minute I hadn't made my decision if I was going to go through with it. My final words to my friend Guy at BK9 were,

"Fuck it, it's not like I'm marrying the girl."

A greater lie has never been spoken, but that's a story for another chapter. She was working until ten o'clock that Saturday night and told me to pick her up on her corner at eleven. I thought it was strange to not pick her up at the house, but she said her brother was there and she didn't want him breaking her chops over who she was leaving the house with at such a late hour. Eleven o'clock came and I sat in my car waiting for her on the corner. When she finally came out, I was instantly happy about my decision. She looked just like she did in the picture. The pretty face, the sweet smile and the great ass. She got in the car and said hello as she scrambled to put her bag down and her seatbelt on. Me, being the charmer I am, decided to tell her she smelled nice. Her response to me was, *"it's called a shower."* Less than one minute in my life and the four words out of her mouth after hello were a smart-ass remark, and it didn't stop there. The whole ride back to Brooklyn and the first two hours sitting on my couch attempting to watch a movie consisted of one wise ass comment after another. I walked outside to smoke a cigarette and call Chris. I told him I couldn't stand her, and I was going to punt her back to Staten Island where she came from. He talked me down attributing her attitude to nerves. Maybe he was right. I decided to give her a chance to tone it down and start the night over. When I went back inside, she was a different person. Maybe it was nerves. We spent the rest of the night watching movies and talking. We stayed up until six in the morning, and after a few hours of sleep, I drove her back to Staten Island. In the department we get every Sunday off plus a rotating day during the week. Every week for the next month we spent the nights before those two days in my apartment, eating pizza, watching movies, and getting to know each other. I liked her a lot. She was so easy to be around and so positive about everything. She made me feel comfortable showing the real me. She was the exact opposite of Julie and that was exactly what I needed.

It didn't go off without a hitch. Julie was still in and out of my life, and out of respect for Diana, I told her I couldn't see her anymore.

It wasn't easy, and she was understandably upset, but it was the right thing to do. I didn't want to be like my father in this situation after seeing the heartache his behavior caused, and if there was going to be a future for us, I had to do things the right way in the present day. Every time I looked at a picture of her smiling my heart would break. She was so good, and so good for me. We stayed in touch, texting back and forth a few times a week, and the truth was that I missed her a lot . In early December of 2010, the saga of me and Julie ended for good. We did what should've been done a year earlier and put our toxic relationship to rest. Diana would come to my house and help me put up my Christmas tree a week later. Our first holiday together was interrupted by the Boxing Day blizzard of 2010, and it wasn't until New Year's Eve that we saw each other again. A chapter of my life had come to an end and a new one was beginning. As 2011 started, the story of my life would include someone new, and a little Sicilian girl from Staten Island named Diana, would show me what true love really was.

CHAPTER 32

Two Weddings and Two Surgeries

With a new girlfriend, almost a year back in meetings and my titration off Suboxone going according to plan, 2011 promised to be my best year in a while. Sure, I was still taking steroids on and off, but at that time in my life I didn't see that as the problem it really was. The Fresh was still my homegroup, but the landscape had somewhat changed. Betty moved to Florida to be with her family, Kevin the Cop had passed away far too young, and after his own valiant battle with cancer, Dougie would pass in the fall of 2010. I was able to see Dougie a few times in that last year, and although I felt like I should've done more, the words his daughter said to me at his funeral, and a letter I would read from him almost a decade later, showed me that he never stopped thinking of me as the son he never had. Although those losses were great, there was still a great group of people at the Fresh. Along with Stevie and Little Chris, some new faces had made their way through the doors over the last couple of years. Three of those people were Little Greggy, Sean, and Anna. Little Greggy got out of long-term treatment at nineteen years old with three years sober. He was one of the nicest kids I ever came across and he was wise beyond his years. Sean and Anna had been coming around for a couple of years, and I never remember them as anything but a couple. Me, Sean, and Anna all separately relapsed and came back around the same time in 2010. Chris, along with Little Greggy took me and Sean through the twelve steps at weekly meets in Chris's apartment. We would read, talk, eat, and play video games, all in the name of getting sober. We would eat together before meetings at the Fresh and hang out after. We all became good friends and valuable support for one another. When I started seeing Diana, they welcomed her with open arms, which meant the world to both of us. She had no idea about the world I was a part of, and no amount of explanation could do it justice. Although she wasn't one of us, their kindness and acceptance made her feel comfortable and helped her fit right in.

My mother's life was changing as well. After many years of being alone, she now had a man in her life. He was old and new, as him and his wife were friends with my parents way back when. I remember him coming by the house all the time when I was a kid and I always liked him. Even after my dad left, he would always come by to make sure me and my mom were ok. His wife had passed away a year earlier and when his mourning period was over, he decided to find my mother. They had lost touch over the years and my mother had since sold her house and moved. One early spring morning when she was walking her dog in Bay Ridge, a car pulled up next to her and a familiar voice called her name. His name was Mario, and he found my mother just like he planned. They talked for a while and made plans to see each other again. From that day on they were inseparable. She was hesitant to tell me of her new situation, but when she told me who it was, I couldn't have been more excited for her. I knew he was a nice guy and it was nice to see my mother happy. As I got to know him my approval of the relationship only grew. Mario was everything my father was, and everything he wasn't. He was a tough guy from the streets of Brooklyn, but he never got involved in the things my father did. He was an honest man that worked hard his whole life to provide for his family. He was handsome and charming just like my father, but he didn't go overboard. He was comfortable in his own skin and didn't need the approval of other people to validate himself. He was one of the funniest men I ever met, and we would spend many an afternoon on his couch having a laugh at the expense of Diana and my Mother. He cared deeply for her and he treated me like a son. For all these reasons I couldn't have been more grateful that he came into her life.

April rolled around and the first of two weddings was about to take place. Sean and Anna were tying the knot and it was the first big event me and Diana were attending as a couple. Diana loved to dance which isn't my strong suit, but that night I didn't care. We danced every song and by the end of the night I could barely walk. The next wedding was in August and it was Chris and Marissa's. It was held at a beautiful beachfront catering hall in Long Island. Me, Greggy, and Sean were all groomsmen, and it turned out to be a beautiful day. As we were all eating, dancing and celebrating the newlyweds, I had another moment of complete gratitude and serenity. I thought to myself ,*this is what it's all about.* At one time or another our lives were in shambles, now, we were living life the way it should be. We were young, sober adults and if we kept on the right path, our futures were without limits. I looked over at Diana, and although we had only known each other a year, I could see us being at that altar one day, with Chris, Sean, Anna and Marissa, celebrating us the same way we celebrated them. All I had to do was stay clean and sober one day at a time and anything was possible.

2011 wasn't all sunshine and rainbows. The Tuesday after Chris's wedding I was scheduled to have surgery on my left foot. In early 2010 my heel started to bother me and I saw a foot doctor to see what the issue was. I was diagnosed with plantar fasciitis and given anti-inflammatory pills and a cortisone shot. This remedy lasted a few months before I had to go back with the same issue. After the fourth time the doctor suggested a surgical procedure to release pressure on the ligament. Between the surgery and physical therapy after, I was looking at a six-week stint on medical leave. I was just looking forward to walking without pain, as the two months leading up to the surgery became less and less bearable, especially at work. My only fear was the possible need for pain meds. I had been good for a year and a half and I was scheduled to come off Suboxone later that month. I didn't want to do anything to mess that up, so I discussed my concerns with both doctors. After weighing the options, we agreed to let the Suboxone doctor take care of pain management. He prescribed me twelve Norco 10/325 and told me to stop taking Suboxone the day before the surgery.

The surgery went off without a hitch. Mario drove me to and from the hospital and Diana stayed with me the first few days to help me around the apartment. The painkillers weren't an issue, as I only took them as prescribed the day after the surgery before following the doctor's instructions and going back on my small dose of Suboxone. I was proud of myself and relieved. The next six weeks went smooth and I was able to return to work in full capacity by early October. I was having trouble getting off the last milligram of Suboxone, so the doctor decided to keep me on for another two months, going down a quarter of a milligram every two weeks. The foot was feeling great so I decided to rejoin my Sunday softball team for the playoff run. In my first at bat of the day I popped a ball up to shallow right field. I dropped the bat, took one step out of the box, and collapsed. The sharpest pain I have ever felt in my life pierced the bottom of my left foot and shot up my whole leg. At first I thought it was a cramp, being the foot hadn't been stretched like that in a few months. When I tried to get up and walk it off, the pain became more intense. My teammates helped me off the field and I spent the rest of the morning with my foot in a cooler of ice, watching the games. The pain got worse as the day went on and when I got home the bottom of the foot had started to bruise. This wasn't the pain I experienced the entire year leading up to my surgery. I knew there was something seriously wrong. I called out from work the next day and went to my foot surgeon. He sent me for an MRI, and the results came back as a partially ruptured plantar fascia. I would need another surgery to repair the damage and it would be more invasive than the last with a longer recovery time. I just made it through one and now I had to go through another. I was down to my last bit of Suboxone, and now that process would be interrupted again. I was frustrated and scared, knowing the the pain would be greater this time around. The doctor, feeling the same, prescribed me thirty Norco 10/325 with the same instructions as before. Take them as needed then go back on Suboxone. He would determine the dose depending on the duration of my time on the Norco. He must've noticed my apprehension, because he assured me that I would be fine if I followed his instructions. It sounded easy enough, but I knew myself. I got off easy the first time because the pain wasn't bad, and I was only on them for a day. The Suboxone was still in my system so the Norco didn't give me a high. Now I was on nothing, a milligram a day. I would be on the pills for a longer period, and there was a good chance the drug would produce the euphoric feeling my mind and body knew all too well. Once that happened, I didn't know if I would be able to control it. The fear was real, and I went into that surgery with a sense of dread.

The surgery took place on November 11th. It went smoothly and Mario picked me up and dropped me off as he did the first time. Diana stayed with me the first two days and helped me around the house just as she did three months earlier. The pain was bad, much worse than the first. I tried taking Ibuprofen and Tylenol, but it didn't work. After three days of torturing myself I took a Norco. Twenty minutes later the euphoria hit and I knew I was in trouble. I loved the feeling. As much as I didn't want to love it, as bad as I knew it was for me, I couldn't help it. I took another one an hour later and by the end of the night I took ten more. Just like that I relapsed again. I finished the bottle by the end of the week and when I called the Suboxone doctor I came clean with him. He put me back on eight milligrams a day and basically told me I was back at day one. He was right, I was back at day one, but nobody else had to know that. I justified my actions on the fact I was in pain. I blamed the doctor, to take the responsibility off myself. The holidays came and I finally met Diana's family. I put on a good front and I fit right in from day one. As 2011 came to an end, the year that started off with such promise, ended in disaster. I would put on a mask and show everyone the Tommy I wanted them to see, but underneath the beast was awake yet again, and I would have to figure out a way to keep it at bay.

CHAPTER 33

2012

Walking in the doors of my first meeting in 2005 was the hardest thing I ever had to do, until I had to walk into the same places five years later counting days again. Humbling myself and doing it for a third time was something I wasn't willing to do, so I kept my relapse a secret. The guilt and shame were bad enough to begin with, and the feelings were only made worse when people would commend me on my strength and courage for getting through two surgeries without overdoing the pain meds. I would never speak at meetings and when people would ask why I wasn't celebrating my anniversaries, I would say I wanted to be off Suboxone first or I want to get past the amount of time I had previously attained before I celebrated again. It was all bullshit. Twelve step recovery is a program of honesty, and I was anything but. After a while I stopped going to meetings. I would stop by the Fresh here and there, but for all intents and purposes, I was once again hiding from the people I knew would see the truth. As time passed, I was spending more time with Donny. He was a great guy, but hanging out with him just furthered my drug use. Oxycontin wasn't around in its original formula anymore so the new industry standard for opiate addicts were called Roxicodone, street term Roxis or Blues. They were small, blue, thirty milligram oxycodone pills with no acetaminophen. It wasn't Oxycontin, but it was the best thing available, and it did the job. They ran anywhere from fifteen to thirty dollars a pill on the street, depending on supply and demand. Donny would get a shitload of them every month from his doctor and sell them in bulk at a discount. It was a nice racket for him, and he would give me twenty or thirty a month for ten dollars a pill. I told him I was selling them for extra money, but I was full of shit. Every time I knew his shipment was coming through, I would stop taking Suboxone for a few days, binge on the Blues for as long as they lasted, then jump back on the Subs, with no one the wiser. It was a vicious hamster wheel that showed no signs of slowing down. There were times I would trade Marco my Suboxone for pills and run out early, getting viciously sick in the process. Speaking from my own experience, Suboxone withdrawal is one of the worst out there. It takes three days to start because of the long half life of the drug, then when it finally kicks in it's miserable. On top of that it lasts forever, the physical part of standard dope sick is three or four days of intense physical effects. Suboxone can last months. I would show up at Donny's looking like death and he would give me Xanax to take the edge off while I waited for my script to be renewed. This process became exhausting and I found myself blaming Suboxone and the doctor who gave it to me. I always shifted the blame elsewhere and now it got to the point of me trying to get off Suboxone by using Xanax and Blues. That never worked and I would always wind up back at the doctor, sick and suffering, asking for another chance with the program.

With all this going on, I continued to keep up personal appearances at work and with the family. My steroid use grew, and I made sure I worked out every day. If I had Suboxone or Blues in my system, my physical appearance gave no indication of my inner struggle. When I was sick, I just stayed in the house or at Donny's until I could get right again. If Diana asked any questions, I just said I had the flu or a stomach virus. All in all, I was holding it together pretty well. One morning in June, I was on a recycling route with one of the old timers in BK9. As I was tossing a bag of bottles out to him, I felt a pinch in my right elbow. I didn't think much of it and we moved on with the route. On the next stop, while tossing another bag, the pinch came again, followed by shooting pain, the complete numbness in my right hand. I immediately knew something was wrong and stopped what I was doing. After a few moments of resting the arm, the symptoms just got worse. I called the supervisor, and in what was becoming an all too familiar occurrence, was transported to the hospital for further examination. After the standard run through at the hospital, visit to the department medical facility and subsequent orthopedic follow up, it was determined to be a pinched nerve in my elbow that would need surgery to repair. I have to be honest, I was happy that I needed surgery. As crazy as it sounds, I knew that I would be home for a few months with a steady supply of painkillers and the excuse to use them. I didn't even bother telling the Suboxone doctor this time around. My prescription loving orthopedic doctor would give me sixty Percocet 10/325 every fourteen days. I know it wasn't his intention for me to go through them the way I was, but as soon as I got them, I would calculate the amount of days that was needed to request a new one. It came out to 4.2 pills a day, which was approximately one every six hours. Without him knowing my history, that seemed reasonable considering the amount of pain I told him I was in.

My surgery took place on August 8th . I was already out on medical leave for two months, and between the surgery, post op healing time and physical therapy, I was looking at another three. It didn't even phase me, as I just viewed it as one less obstacle in the way of me doing what I wanted to do. Diana drove me to the hospital the day of the surgery and everything went well. While we were waiting for my discharge papers, we received some great news. Her brother Nicky's wife Jen had just given birth to their first son Nicholas. There was a new addition to the family and Diana was bursting at the seems wanting to go see him. We left the hospital and headed home. After getting my medication and various snacks for the evening, I told her I was ok to be alone. She didn't want to leave me, but I knew she wanted to go see her newborn nephew. I broke her chops about it for months after, but I was perfectly ok with being left alone with my tv, my snacks, and my Percocet. I didn't see it at the time, but that night was the catalyst for the heights my addiction would eventually reach.

I woke up on my couch early the next afternoon. There was water all over the floor and crushed potato chips all over the couch. There were cigarette ashes everywhere and there were holes burnt in my shorts. When I looked to my left, the bottle of Percocet I filled the day before had twelve pills left. When I did the math in my head that left forty-eight pills missing. It should've shocked me, and I should've seen it as a sign I was out of control. Instead, I compared the milligram count to my Oxycontin days and convinced myself it wasn't that bad. Being in a pretty good deal of pain at this point, I took a handful of what I had left and called Donny. I knew I would need more. I had Suboxone for dope sickness, but that wasn't going to help the pain in my arm. He quickly brought me twenty blues of his own and a handful of Xanax, telling me to make it last because he wasn't getting more for a couple of weeks. Marco scored me fifty Vicodin 5/500's and I was once again flush with what I needed. A week later I followed up with the surgeon and got another script for Percocet. A week after that I got more Blues and Xanax from Donny. I was in full blown relapse mode and without anything holding me in check, things were about to take another bad turn.

I never experienced Benzo withdrawal in the past as my use of the drugs were limited to certain situations. I never took them consistently for a long enough period or in a high enough dose for my body to become dependent on them. I had been taking between six and eight milligrams of Xanax for the two weeks after the surgery on top of a shitload of pain medication. I woke up one day out of Xanax and didn't really think twice about it until a few hours later. When I described Suboxone withdrawal I said I would take dope sick over it every day and twice on Sundays. I would take all that and a bat to the face over Benzo withdrawal. It is by far the worst thing I ever felt in my life. Your whole body shakes, you can't breathe, your heart races, you can't focus, and every step you take feels like it's going to be the last one before your whole body gives out and you die. That's how I felt that morning and no amount of Percocet, Vicodin or Suboxone would make it go away. It was the worst anxiety I ever felt times two hundred. It got so bad I just sat curled on my couch crying. Diana was freaking out as she had never seen me like this before. I called Donny and told him what was going on and he told me it was withdrawal from the Xanax. I asked him for more, but he was out, and it would be hours before he could get any. I called my mother hysterically crying and told her I was having a bad anxiety attack. It had been a long time since I went to her for this. I can only imagine her being brought back to the early 2000's when this was a weekly occurrence. She agreed to take me to her doctor, but I had to pick her up. Driving was going to be difficult, but I needed something to make this go away. I sucked it up and we made the trip to her doctor's office in downtown Brooklyn. I was in bad shape and the wait was excruciating. On top of being strung out on painkillers and if full blown withdrawal from Xanax, the amount of drugs I had taken over the last two weeks messed up my body functions and my body had been retaining urine the last few days. I spent the hour-long wait squirming in my chair and in the bathroom, standing in front of the toilet bowl with my hand under running water trying desperately to empty my bladder and make the burning pain in my abdomen stop. Shortly before I was called in to see the doctor, I was finally able to go and the relief I felt was amazing. I went into the exam room and told her what she needed to hear. She prescribed me Valium and referred me to a Psychiatrist. She didn't know any better. All she knew was that her patient, and friend's son, was suffering. She didn't know my history with addiction, so much like Dr. Fred a decade earlier, she treated me for what I presented. I went home that night and took some Valium and felt better twenty minutes later. I saw the psychiatrist a week later and was prescribed one milligram of Klonipin twice a day. I spent the next two months rehabbing my elbow. I cut the daily use of painkillers and was back on the Suboxone program. I was back in the gym and back on Testosterone. The outside looked good again and I put the two-week binge after my surgery out of my mind. I got to meet little Nicholas and it was love at first sight, he was adorable, and I was looking forward to getting closer with Diana's family. I returned to work on October 28th one day before Hurricane Sandy hit. I would spend the next two months helping the people of Brooklyn and Staten Island clean up the wreckage of the devastating storm. Day after day we would go to houses, put peoples entire life into the back of a garbage truck and haul it away. The hardest part was them thanking us for doing it. I would often go home at night and be overcome with emotion, thinking about the lives that were so greatly affected by the events that October day. I dealt with these feelings, along with my growing internal struggle by taking more and more Klonipin. By early 2013 I talked the doctor up to the maximum daily dose of the drug which was two milligrams, three times a day. It wasn't about getting high anymore, it was about not feeling at all. I buried the guilt and buried the shame. I didn't even think of my sober life anymore. This was how it was now, and I would try to make the best of it. Good on the outside, dead on the inside, is how I would carry on in the days, months, and years ahead.

CHAPTER 34

Some Days Are Better Than Others

While 2013 was a largely uneventful year, 2014 was anything but. My use of Klonipin was increasing to the point of me struggling to make it through an entire month without running out of my prescription. I was maintaining my opiate use with Suboxone daily, and one or two binges a month on Blues, Percs or Vicodin. I was injecting four hundred milligrams of Testosterone a week, in three-month cycles, with a short break in between each. My relationship with Diana was going well and aside from a few isolated incidences, I was showing up to work on a consistent basis. From the outside looking in, my life appeared to be going as well as could be.

It was a Saturday morning in early February, and the day started like any other. I woke up at four in the morning, got dressed, took a Suboxone, two Klonipin, drank a Red Bull, and headed to work. Halfway through the ride, as I was sitting at a red light, I was rear ended by a guy who was texting while driving. The force of the impact caused my head to snap forward and back into the headrest, knocking me unconscious for a short period of time. I was transported to the hospital to rule out any major injuries, and when all was said and done, I was diagnosed with bruising to my shoulder and chest, and a mild concussion. My car, on the other hand, wasn't so lucky, sustaining over ten thousand dollars in damage. With my lease a month away from expiring and Mario's son overseeing the local dealerships maintenance department, I was able to get it repaired and returned with no issues.

The insurance took care of my rental and I was able to lease a new car a month later. The head trauma was worse than originally thought, and I suffered from post-concussion symptoms for months following the accident. I had severe headaches every day and struggled to keep my balance at times. My vision would get blurry, and there were days I had to sit in the dark for hours at a time, while the symptoms subsided. I was out of work for five months and it was suggested that I sue the person that hit me. At first, I was hesitant, but after suffering through that first month I decided to consult with a lawyer recommended by a guy at work. With no broken bones or disfiguring facial injuries he didn't think I had much of a case, but as a favor to my friend, he was willing to investigate it for me. I returned to work in July, and lost track of the situation, figuring nothing would come out of it. A few weeks later I got a call from the lawyer. Much to the surprise of both of us, the rental company agreed to settle my case for twenty-five thousand dollars. After lawyer fees I walked away with almost seventeen thousand. It was a nice little windfall, and I was grateful for how it all turned out, but as my addiction was progressing, I knew deep down, that money was like putting a loaded gun in my hands.

The feeling of happiness I got from winning my lawsuit was quickly overshadowed by a call I received from my mother, in the early morning hours of Monday, August 11th, 2014. My Uncle woke up to find my cousin Denis lying lifeless in the bathtub. There were high levels of his drug of choice, PCP, in his system, which ultimately led to a brain aneurysm, that was the official cause of death. At thirty-three years old, my cousin had lost his lifelong battle with addiction. I was deeply saddened, but I wasn't shocked at all. My cousin, like me, had been flirting with death his entire adolescent and adult life. Jails, institutions and death are the three outcomes of untreated addiction, and he paid the ultimate price. We developed a strong bond in the time between my aunt dying and me getting sober. I tried to sway him in the same direction, but when he continued his path, I had to stop hanging around him, only seeing him occasionally at a family gathering. It was the right thing to do for my sobriety in those early days, but nine years later, being in full blown relapse mode, I couldn't see that. All I could see in my head was my cousin, as the little kid who just wanted a normal home, and parents who loved him. My uncle tried to be that later in his life, and he took care of my cousin the best way he could, but the damage was already done. I always said he never stood a chance, but that's a lie. There's always a chance, and in the aftermath of his death, I felt that I was his chance and I failed him. The feelings were real, but who was I kidding ? At any given moment it could be me in the box right along with him. I couldn't help myself, so how would I ever have helped him? I spent the entire night of the wake conversing with his friends and my family about the life he led, and how it killed him one minute, then out in my car sniffing Roxis and Klonipin the next. We buried my cousin on a Wednesday morning and life continued, just as it always does. His death should've been a wakeup call, but it was the complete opposite. I didn't want to cope with my feelings, so I once again did what I knew how to do, I got high and numbed it all away.

Over the next two months, I spent ten-thousand dollars on painkillers. I got them on the cheap from Donny, and when those ran out, I got them from Marco's connection for regular street prices. At one point, me and my friend Devin got a deal on two hundred Roxis. If I just sold half of my cut at regular street price I could've at least broke even. Instead, I ate all my half, and bought Devin's half back from him and ate all of those. One morning on my route, I found a bottle of cough medicine with hydrocodone in it and took it home with me. The plan was to spend my Sunday getting high and watching baseball. Diana was heading to work at one o'clock, so around eleven, I mixed half the bottle of the cough syrup with a twenty-ounce Sprite and chugged it down within fifteen minutes. It hit me hard and I must've passed out on the couch. When Diana woke me up to say goodbye, I couldn't see a thing. I was high as a kite and completely blind. I didn't say anything to Diana. I just gave her a kiss goodbye and told her I'd see her later. As time slowly moved, nothing changed. My vision was gone, and I started to panic. I thought to myself, *I finally went too far.* After all the years of drinking and drugging, a bottle of cough medicine was going to do me in, and I would live the rest of my life blind. My life would be altered forever and in that moment I pleaded with God to help me. *I swear if you give me back my sight, I will straighten my life out for good,* were the words that came out of my mouth. After an hour or so my sight started to improve. The darkness became cloudiness, then the cloudiness became fuzzy, then the fuzziness became a lack of focus. Finally my sight came back in full. From start to finish the whole process lasted about four hours. It was the longest, scariest four hours of my life, and I felt an overwhelming rush of relief and gratitude when it was over. God answered my prayers, and I knew I was lucky. I was so happy, and so grateful, that I decided to celebrate by mixing the rest of the bottle with another Sprite, and doing it all over again. This time I just did it slower so I wouldn't go blind again. That day epitomized how far my addiction had progressed. I wasn't robbing anyone, I wasn't collecting cans for crack money. I wasn't writing my own prescriptions or running drug money for Russian criminals and I wasn't drinking or doing cocaine. I was showing up to work and paying my bills. I was in good physical shape and people wanted to be around me. All those things made it easy to justify what I was doing, but that day showed that I was just as bad, if not worse than I was ten years earlier.

I called out of work the next day because I was physically shot from the whole experience. As I sat on my couch taking stock of my life, I came to the conclusion that I had to stop what I was doing before I lost everything, but I wanted to do it my way. I decided that I would go back on Suboxone full time, and do it the right way, decreasing every month until I was completely off. Once I got off that, I would wean myself off the Klonipin and I would be done with all the bullshit once and for all. I also decided to buy Diana an engagement ring. I knew I wanted her in my life and even though I was in no shape to get married, I didn't want to let her slip away. I spent a few weeks shopping around before finding the perfect ring. I paid for most of it with the money I had left over from the lawsuit, and I put the rest on a credit card. As December rolled around, I was sticking to my Suboxone program and I wasn't overdoing the Klonipin. I felt good, I felt optimistic, and on December 5th, 2014, with the lights turned down low, and the Staind song Tangled up in You playing in the background, I got down on one knee in the living room of my apartment, and asked Diana to marry me. She said yes, and now the plan was complete. By this time next year, I planned to be fully clean and sober. I planned to save enough money to have our wedding in 2016, and I could put all the insanity behind me once and for all. That was my plan, but it wasn't the plan for me.

Rest In Peace
Denis S. Doyle
7/4/81 – 8/11/14

CHAPTER 35

Vaporized and Relocated

Shortly after I proposed to Diana in December, I began to develop a moderate burning pain in my back. I brushed it off as the usual aches and pains of the daily grind of the job and didn't think much of it, but as days went on it only got worse. Along with the pain came difficulty urinating, and after a visit to the ER, it was suggested I see a urologist. At this point, my nerves started to take over, and I spent night after night googling my symptoms. Everything pointed to a prostate issue and considering my abundant steroid use over the last few years, I immediately assumed I had cancer. The whole situation was the perfect excuse for me to go right back down the same rabbit hole I spent the past three months trying to get out of. I didn't want to deal with the feelings I was having so I started taking Klonipin by the handful, and I ran through my January script of ninety, 2MG pills in less than a week. Marco sold me his Xanax script, and I ran through them in three days. I bought half of my friend Justin's Valium script and went through them in a week. It was less than halfway through the month and I had no benzos. The withdrawal started coming on strong, so I reached out to Donny and he got me forty Xanax sticks. He told me the neighborhood was dry and his pills weren't coming until the end of the month, so I had to make them last. My mother still had some connections in the medical field and she was able to get me an appointment with a Urologist within a week.

I arrived at the Urologist office in downtown Brooklyn at six in the evening. Mario, my mother, and Diana came with me for support.

Between the pills and the worsening symptoms of whatever was wrong with me, I could barely get out of bed. I went through a few tests that first appointment, and he didn't like what he saw. My prostate was severely enlarged and because of that, I couldn't empty my bladder. He quickly gave me some medication to try to shrink the prostate, along with ordering a battery of the most uncomfortable tests known to man. At the worst point, I was measuring my urine in a blender cup, often building up over a liter before I was able to urinate. Less than two weeks after my first appointment with the urologist I was scheduled for an emergency TUVP, or Trans Urethral Vaporization Process. They couldn't shrink the prostate fast enough and the amount of urine being retained was at a dangerous level, causing the doctor to fear permanent kidney damage if we didn't act quick. They needed to create a lane for the urine to empty from the bladder and vaporizing a hole through the prostate was the best way to do so. In the early evening hours of February 3rd, 2015, I woke up in a recovery room in Methodist Hospital in Brooklyn. The surgery went off without a hitch, but I had to be kept overnight for observation.

Normal people worry about normal things when they go for surgery, like recovery time or possible complications, but I couldn't care less about any of that. My biggest worry was how many benzos I needed to get me through the night and if they were going to give me enough pain meds to keep me well. The pain meds weren't an issue. They gave me a double dose along with the anesthesia to break through the Suboxone. When I woke up in recovery, they gave me a shot of morphine, followed by a Percocet every four hours. That was enough to keep me more than well. Along with that, I stashed a bottle of Xanax sticks in my bag to get me through the night. Once everyone left, and the doctors and nurse visits slowed to a trickle, I was finally able to throw back a few sticks to mix with the pain meds. As uncomfortable as I was, the mixture of my two favorite drugs was enough to make it somewhat bearable. I slipped in and out of consciousness the rest of the night, eagerly awaiting the pending removal of the catheter that was placed in me after the surgery. At eight o'clock the next morning, the doctor came in to do the deed. He told me he was going to quickly remove the tube in one felt swoop. In his exact words, it was like ripping off a band aid and all I had to do was push out like I was trying to take a massive shit. He hit three, and I pushed out. Every story I was told about this process was horrific. Maybe it was all the Xanax I ate overnight, mixed with the pain meds, but it wasn't bad at all. The next step is where the problem came. In order to leave the hospital, I needed to show them I could urinate on my own. If I couldn't they would have to send me home catheterized and that was the last thing I wanted. I went in the bathroom fully expecting to go with no issue. After an hour, there was nothing, and now I started to develop a sharp stabbing pain in my pelvic area. It got to the point I couldn't even stand up. My mother of all people was asking them to give me pain meds. I was in so much pain, I was now begging to get the catheter put back in, anything to make the pain stop was fine with me. Just as the nurse came and stuck me with a shot of morphine, the Physicians Assistant came in with a catheter. As soon as he put it in the tip of my penis I felt like a dam was broken. I quickly told him to take it out and I ran into the bathroom and took the best piss of my life. The problem wasn't with my prostate or bladder. There was a small clot of blood in the way, and as soon as it was broken, I was good to go. I was good to go and now I was high as a kite. The shot of morphine hit me like a ton of bricks. I told myself heading into this surgery that I would go right back on Suboxone when I got home. That shot changed everything. I got home and immediately scored a bunch of Roxis from Donny. I called the doctor and told him I was in a lot of pain and he prescribed me sixty Perc 10's. I tried to go back to work in the middle of March but it was too soon. Hitting one big bump in the truck caused me to start urinating blood, and after meeting with my doctor and the Department medical staff I was placed on modified duty. With nothing to do but go to work, answer phones all day and come home, my use of painkillers and benzos increased more and more with each passing week. One day I was out of Percs and suboxone and everyone I called was dry. I couldn't get anything so I called Donny and lied to him, telling him my friend wanted heroin. Donny was much like my cousin Denis in one respect. My cousin would drink, smoke weed and sniff coke with me, but he drew the line at Angel Dust. I believe it was because he struggled with it so much, he didn't want me to go down that road with him. Donny would get me Xanax and Roxis all the time, but I knew he would draw the line at heroin. As crazy as it sounds Donny still considered me clean, and because of his own struggles with heroin, I knew he wouldn't want me going down that path. The lie worked and he got me a bundle. For years I justified my drug use by saying it was all prescribed. I even told myself it was ok taking other peoples pills because my doctor didn't give me enough and I was only taking them for the crippling anxiety I would get without them. The crippling anxiety was just withdrawal, but I still convinced myself otherwise. The moment I picked my head up from the bathroom sink and looked in the mirror after snorting two lines of heroin, was the moment I stopped believing myself. That was the day I finally accepted that I was in full blown active addiction. It was that day that all the lies I had been telling myself came to light. I finally saw it for what it was, and the truth was I didn't even want to stop.

April rolled around and Diana's brother and sister-in-law were about to have their second child. Needing more room for their new addition they decided to buy their first home. I made no secret about how much I loved their apartment and I always told them to let me know if they ever left. When her brother called me to tell me the news, I jumped on the opportunity. I drove out to Staten Island and met with the landlords, who were a couple of the nicest people I ever met. They told me they would raise the rent fifty dollars from what they were charging Nicky and Jen but would never raise it after that. To this day that promise has been kept. I gave them my deposit and made my way back to Brooklyn. On May 1st I would finally make the move most of Brooklyn had made already. Staten Island would be good for me, it was a nicer apartment in a nicer neighborhood. Donny had gotten locked up for violating a restraining order and he was really my only friend in the neighborhood. I was paying street value for everything now, dealing exclusively with Marco and his people. I figured the farther I got away from that whole crew, the better. I thought I would slow down. I thought I would be able to tame the beast, but wherever I went there I was. It was only a matter of time before I found a whole new way of getting what I needed.

CHAPTER 36

Crashing Through The Door

I tried to spend as little time as possible in Brooklyn. I thought the less time I spent in the old neighborhood, the better. Echoing the words of Brinsley one more time, it didn't take long to find what I needed in my new surroundings. The process of getting pills became exhausting. I had a psychiatrist for Klonipin, a doctor for Suboxone, and my orthopedic for Percocet. One was in Staten Island and two were on the opposite ends of Brooklyn. I had to use three different pharmacies because no legitimate one would fill all three of those drugs. In a matter of three months, this whole process became consolidated to one doctor on Staten Island. I would call him Dr. Webster because of his resemblance to the Emanuel Lewis character on the old 80's sitcom. His office was in the basement of a small medical building on the North Shore of the island, and one look at the clientele would give you an immediate idea of what was going on behind those closed doors. On my first visit, I explained my history with opiate use and that I just moved to the Island and didn't want to go back and forth to Brooklyn for my Suboxone. Without hesitation he wrote me a script for double the amount I asked for. There was no urine test and no asking for my records from the previous doctor, just a quick, easy stroke of his pen and I had what I needed. Between that day and my next visit, I was informed by my Psychiatrist that he was moving to Houston for family reasons. He gave me the number of a colleague on the Island to continue my treatment and wished me luck. I spent three years training this guy to give me the max dose of Klonipin without any hesitation, on every visit. Five minutes a month and I had my script. The minute I stepped into the new doctors office I knew that wasn't going to be the case. She wrote me the script I needed, but then she interrogated me about everything. She wanted to know why I was on such a high dose and why I had been on it for so long. She wanted my medical history, and any history of drug and alcohol use. She wanted monthly drug tests and immediately started drawing up a plan to taper me off the Klonipin. Long story short, that was the last time I went to see her. With no legal way to get my Klonipin, I figured I'd ask Dr. Webster. I knew it was a long shot because it's hard to get a doctor to give a benzo and an opiate together, but I thought I'd give it a shot. I couldn't have been more wrong. I explained that my psychiatrist moved, and I had no way of getting what I needed. All he wanted to see was a bottle of a previous script and once I showed him he wrote away. Just like that I had a one stop shop for all my prescription needs, or at least two of the three. I still needed to see the orthopedic for my Percocet, at least until the following month. I did it once so why not try again. I showed Dr. Webster my script for Percocet and asked if he could write the same amount for me to avoid the trip to Brooklyn, the same story I used for the Suboxone. After a brief hesitation, he wrote me a script, but not for sixty Perc 10's. He wrote me a script for sixty Roxi 30's. I filled the Suboxone and Klonipin at my regular pharmacy in Brooklyn, then filled the Roxis in Staten Island and paid with cash to avoid any red flags on my insurance. Dr. Webster became the best drug dealer I ever had. While the process became easier, my addiction just got worse. I still needed to go outside of my own script for my benzo intake and would trade my surplus of Suboxone for Xanax and Valium. I would go through the sixty Roxis in a few days, then spend the rest of the month taking Suboxone. I never got sick and I never got desperate. It was a drug addicts dream scenario. What I did get with each passing day was a greater feeling that I would never be able to stop what I was doing, and with that came feelings of guilt and shame that were just as bad as they were ten years earlier.

Dominick Vincent was born on May 15, 2015 and we were asked to be his Godparents. I was truly honored, but deep down I knew I didn't deserve it. What kind of role model would I be for this kid if I kept going down the road I was going ? I really should've said no, but then I would have to give them a reason and the only reason I could give was that I wasn't worthy of such an honor because I was a drug addict. If I did that, everyone would know my secret and I couldn't let that happen. I accepted and much like everything else, I would figure out a way to do it high. It was August 2, 2015, the day of Dom's Christening and the weather was beautiful. By now the amount of benzos I was taking was having a severe effect on my memory. I would black out for days at a time and often not remember what I did or how I did it. Because of the pill intake and my continued use of steroids, my recovery from the prostate surgery was taking forever. I was still on modified duty and it got to the point of the doctor putting me on medication to strengthen my bladder. He told me this was the last resort, and if it didn't work there was a chance I would have to use a catheter for the rest of my life. Looking back, all I needed to do was stop the pills and stop the steroids. It was as simple as that, but in the moment you don't use reason or logic. It was easier for me to use my condition as an excuse to get high. On the day of the christening I spent half the time in the bathroom trying to pee and the other half trying to stay awake so I could give my speech. I have been told the speech was great, and the party was a beautiful celebration of Dominick. Unfortunately, the only way I can remember that day is by looking at photos. I don't remember what I said or how I said it. I don't remember the church ceremony. I don't remember the restaurant we went to or the people I spoke to that day. I only see the pictures, and when I look at them I see a different person. I see distress and unhappiness. I see pain and anger. My eyes were dead and I never smiled. As a matter of fact if you look at any pictures of me from 2012 through 2015, I am never smiling in any of them. It was starting to become noticeable to others, especially on that day, but they chalked it up to the recovery from the surgery, which was an easy excuse for me to use whenever anyone voiced their concerns.

A few weeks after the christening, the medication for the bladder started to work. After seven long months I was finally able to fully empty my bladder every time I urinated, and it didn't take me a half hour to do so. The whole experience made taking a normal piss something I will never take for granted again. Now that I was functioning normally in that area, it was time to get back to work full duty. I was happy to be back on the truck and on my route. I missed the people, I missed the activity and I missed working with my partner day in and day out. As good as it was to be back, I was a mess. I had no business driving the truck and thankfully my partner liked to do most of the driving. I limited myself to the house to house moving of the vehicle on the route. This would lead to issues if my partner was off, but in that case, I would just volunteer to do most of the loading myself, something that goes over very well with most guys. If my partner for the day wouldn't cooperate, I would just drink an extra red bull or take an Adderall, my newest addition to my ever-growing cocktail of prescription meds, to make myself more alert. I was playing a dangerous game with dangerous equipment and I thank God to this day that I never hurt or killed myself or anyone else.

When I went to see Dr. Webster in October, he looked stressed out. The way he normally wrote scripts was just by looking at the previous month and copying whatever he had written. Normally, there was no drug test, no examination and very limited conversation. This time was different. As soon as I walked in I was asked to pee in a cup. After that he came in and gave me a thorough exam and asked me a laundry list of questions about why I was using the medications he was prescribing, almost like he was being forced to do so. When all was said and done, he told me he could no longer give me Roxis, and he would have to cease the Klonipin the following month. He must've had a lot of heat on him considering the amount of drugs he was giving me multiplied by who knows how many other people for whom he was doing the same. I was in no position to argue and honestly, I was tired of living how I was. If I had the Suboxone I would be ok as far as the opiates. As far as the benzos, I took this as a sign from God, and an opportunity to wean myself off them for good. He gave me the script, and I spent the next thirty days weening myself off the Klonipin. By the time my next visit came around I was completely off the drug, and because I did it gradually, the withdrawal wasn't terrible. There was still some shakiness and rebound anxiety, but nothing I couldn't handle. People noticed an improvement in my appearance and mood almost immediately, and it was nice to be present in my life for the first time in a long time. I wasn't taking any opiates other that Suboxone, and I was feeling so good that I decided it was finally time to come off, so I made my own tapering plan. If all went well, I would be off everything by the New Year.

November went well, and the shakiness from the benzo withdrawal subsided to the point of being almost unnoticeable. I tapered from sixteen milligrams of Suboxone a day to four and I walked into Dr. Webster's office on the Monday before Thanksgiving ready to tell him that this would in fact be my last visit. He looked more relaxed than he had the last two times I saw him and we had a pleasant conversation about his wife, kids, grandkids, his plans for the holiday. Before I could tell him of my progress with my taper and my plans to discontinue our visits, he looked down at my chart and flipped the pages back. In his soft, accented voice he read the words,

" *Suboxone – Eight times two, Oxycodone – Thirty times two, and Klonipin Two times three.* "

He either forgot our conversation two months earlier or didn't care anymore. In that moment I had a decision to make and without hesitation I said yes. I took the scripts and left the office. I dropped the Roxi script off then drove to Brooklyn to fill the other two. When I got in the car with the Klonipin, I opened the bottle and washed down ten of them with a twelve-ounce Red Bull. I drove back to Staten Island, picked up my Roxis, went home, and sniffed five of them in fifteen minutes. Two months of being good, being hopeful, and being present, were gone in a matter of two hours. The rush I got when he wrote me those scripts put me into a blackout. My brain went into overdrive to get what it wanted, and now here I was a few hours later, sitting on my couch right back at square one, almost like I had no control over my actions once that opportunity arose, and that was the scariest part. A week later while coming out of the bathroom stall at work, someone pulled a Xanax stick out of their pocket and offered it to me and I took it without a second thought.

For years my addiction was beating the door down trying to take over my life completely. As bad as it was during certain periods, I maintained some semblance of normalcy by never opening the door all the way. It was a struggle every day and I was losing the battle. I look back on the day at Dr. Websters and the following week in the bathroom at work as the days the door finally came crashing in. I couldn't hold it shut anymore, and I went on a hard two month run that bled into the new year. I was buying two hundred Xanax and thirty Adderall a week on top of my scripts. I also started drinking again, at first it was beer, Sam Adams Winter Lager to be exact, then it was Nyquil. Nyquil was easier to hide, and the combination of alcohol and cough suppressant mixed with everything else I was taking produced the effect I was chasing in a much quicker way. I walked around in a drug and alcohol induced blackout for the entire stretch, not remembering much of what happened. I started putting myself in bad situations, meeting dealers in public places at all hours, even driving a friend around the projects for his cocaine, just so I could get half of his Xanax script. During a two-week vacation in January me and Diana went to Atlantic City for a few days. I remember checking in and eating dinner the first night there, but that's all I remember. The worst part is that I don't remember driving there or back. It was the darkest place my life had gotten to since the night I held a shotgun under my chin over a decade before and those thoughts started to cross my mind once again.

I was due back at work on January 24th. That day was the first and only time I went AWOL from my job. Winter Storm Jonas had just dropped almost twenty-eight inches of snow on the city and I knew I couldn't operate snow equipment in the condition I was in, so I just ignored the phone calls and stayed home. The next day I called out sick because I didn't want to work the shift they had me assigned to. I was running low on Xanax so I called my dealer for ninety pills. My plan was to get a doctor's note for the sick day, then pick up the pills. I shoveled Diana out of her parking spot so she could go to work, then got in my car to drive to the doctors office. As I adjusted the rearview mirror and caught a glimpse of my reflection, I dreaded what I saw. My skin was pale and my gaze was empty. Much like the night in my mother's bedroom over a decade earlier, there was no life left in me and I was utterly defeated. It was in that moment I knew I was done. I didn't want to keep living how I was, but I couldn't stop. I tried so many times only to wind up worse off than before. The next thing I remember is sitting on my couch and dialing the phone. I decided to call my friend John. He was the first person I met when I walked into BK9 on September 9, 2006 to introduce myself two days before my first official shift. We became close over the years eventually realizing we were in the same graduating class in Xaverian many years before. John had his own issues with painkillers after a major back surgery and I spent many nights talking him through his own struggles. I knew he would understand and I knew he would point me in the right direction. The phone rang a few times before the voice on the other end finally came through.

"What's up Dude?" John said in his patented, laid back Bill and Ted-like voice.
"I need help man, I can't stop."

I let it all out, choking back tears through the whole conversation, and he did exactly what I thought he would. He listened, he understood, and he called the departments counseling unit for me. I went the next day and told them my story. They told me I would have to go to detox and rehab. At that point I would've said yes to anything, so I agreed to go away for twenty-eight days and the arrangements were made. A car would pick me up the next day at eleven thirty in the morning and January 27, 2016 would be the start of my new journey into recovery.

CHAPTER 37

You Got That Sparkle Back

I opened my eyes and was confused by my surroundings. This wasn't my house, but for the life of me I couldn't remember where I was. I got up to go to the bathroom and it was as unfamiliar as the moment I opened my eyes a few short minutes before. I knew what was going on. Ever since I was in the Psych Ward fourteen years ago, I would have this recurring dream that I was back there. I would go to the bathroom in the unfamiliar place then realize where I was when I came back out and panned around the room. It was usually then, that I would wake up in my own bed relieved that it was just a dream. I finished up and washed my hands, splashing some cold water on my face so I could get a better look at what was outside the bathroom. When I walked out into the main room I looked around and it was just like the dream. The room was a little different, but the feeling was the same. I walked back to the bed and laid down. I dozed off for what seemed to be a few seconds only to be woken up by a young woman taking my blood pressure, telling me I had to speak to a doctor to discuss my course of treatment. I quickly realized this wasn't a dream. I remembered where I was and I remembered why I was there. I was in a treatment facility about thirty miles outside Philadelphia. I was there because I didn't want to suffer anymore. I didn't want to live with the guilt and shame that controlled my life ever since I took that pill over seven years earlier. I knew I had to change, but at this point in my life I didn't know if I could. I needed help and this place would at least start me in the right direction. I knew from experience, that all I needed was honesty, open mindedness and willingness. If I had that everything else would fall into place.

I was three days into my month long stay and things were moving along well. I was actively participating in all group activities. I was raising my hand and sharing in meetings and I was going out of my way to acquaint myself with the rest of the community. If the rest of the stay were like this, the month would be over in no time and I would be able to go home and start my new life. Day four is when that all changed. With the massive amount of benzos I was taking and the half life of Suboxone being much longer than that of a regular opiate my body had enough in it to keep me out of withdrawal those first few days. On day four the remnants of what was left in my system had run out and I quickly went into full blown withdrawal from both Benzos and Suboxone. I knew it was coming, but the severity at which it came was something I was not at all prepared for. They tried to keep me as comfortable as possible, giving me antihistamines and blood pressure medication to calm my system and melatonin to help me sleep at night. At the end of the day there's only so much they can give. Other than being put into a coma for the duration of the process, this was something I was going to have to go through if I wanted to see the other side. I had muscle aches and nausea from the Suboxone and the benzo withdrawal was exactly like I remembered, only much more intense. My hands shook so uncontrollably at times that my counselor would have to write for me during small group exercises. I couldn't eat, I couldn't sleep, and I couldn't breathe. Every step I took was so unsteady that I thought each one would be my last. My eyes shook when I closed them and the one night I did manage to fall asleep, I woke up shaking violently yet unable to move on my own, something that I found out later on, was a seizure. I entered treatment weighing one hundred and seventy-three pounds. At the height of my detox I was down to one hundred thirty-eight. Anything I looked at for more than a few seconds became distorted and whenever I tried to speak I couldn't get the words to come out to come out the right way. My face was sunken in and my skin was gray. When I used the pay phone to call Diana or my mother, I couldn't look at the reflection staring back at me. I wouldn't let anyone visit me and after a while I even limited the phone calls. I was in the worst physical, mental and emotional state I had ever been, often thinking that my brain was broken and I would never be the same. I would try to make light of the situation, telling my counselors I would be the only person in history that leaves rehab in worse shape than the day I got there. Through it all I knew I still needed to be present. As hard as it was, I managed to make it to every group, every meeting and every meal. I couldn't eat and it was hard for me to participate. Most of the time I just sat there rocking back and forth trying to keep myself together, but I still went. Every night I would sit up in my bed praying for it to end yet every morning it would still be there, the intensity never letting up. On February 10th I was called down to the directors office after dinner and told to call Diana. She answered the phone and told me that my Uncle Denis had passed away earlier that day. He had been sick for a while so it wasn't a surprise, but that didn't make it any easier. He was someone I looked up to and enjoyed being around my whole life. I wish I had the chance to say goodbye to him, but that wasn't meant to be. When that call ended I was faced with a decision. The wake was in five days and they wanted to know if I wanted a day pass to attend the services. For the next three days I struggled back and forth knowing how much my family would want me there, but also knowing I was in no condition to leave treatment. I didn't want to get high. Getting high was the farthest thing from my mind. What I didn't want to do was feel the way I was feeling. I knew if I left treatment, even for a day, I would take something to make the withdrawal go away and whether I liked it or not, that action would more than likely lead me down a path I wouldn't be able to come back from. With a heavy heart and a lump in my throat, I called my mother and told her I wouldn't be able to attend my uncle's funeral. It hurt me as I'm sure it hurt my family, but I needed to do what was right for me and my recovery. As bad as I felt about my choice, I knew my uncle would've understood. That decision was the turning point of my stay in treatment.

In the days that followed I was able to get more and more sleep. At first it was an hour, then two, then three, then finally a whole night. My heart slowed down and my breathing came easier. My hands shook less, and I was able to process my thoughts and words with less and less effort. My appetite came back with a vengeance and I started to put some weight back on. I was able to become a more active member in the community, even agreeing to stay an extra week to make up for the time I couldn't fully participate in my treatment process during my detox. I was able to look back on things in my life and feelings I had that I never knew effected me the way they did. I was able to look back at my first stint in recovery and see the glaring red flags that popped up before my relapse ever happened. I was able to do all this without the outside noise. I wasn't worried about the debt I was in. I wasn't worried about the job or my relationship with Diana. I wasn't worried about how people would look at me when I got home. I just focused on me, knowing that all those other things would work themselves out one way or another and whatever the outcome I would be able to handle it if I stayed clean and sober. The night before I was set to leave, I was asked by the counselors to speak at the "almost alumni" meeting. I sat up on the stage and shared my story with a room full of people I lived with for the last thirty-five days. Being in a room with a bunch of people from Pennsylvania that broke my balls for over a month because I was from New York, I had to open with the fact I was a Met, Cowboy and Ranger fan. My intro was met by a round of boos and heckling you would come to expect from a bunch of Philly fans, but once I got into my story you could've heard a pin drop. I spoke for a half hour and when I was done the whole room applauded. People came to me afterward to talk to me, many of them telling me how much they related to my story. It was a fitting end to my five week stay and I was confident that if I took what I learned there and continued to work on myself when I got home, my future could be as bright as I wanted it to be. As I was filling out my discharge papers the following day, the clinical director passed me in the hallway. It was the same lady who did my intake five weeks earlier. She hugged me, looked in my eyes and said.

"Would you look at that. You got your sparkle back."

Rest In Peace
Denis "Denny" Doyle
9/7/38 – 2/10/16

CHAPTER 38

Recovery

As we stood in the kitchen, talking about life in general, my father-in-law grabbed something out of the cabinet and walked in my direction. He had gone to the doctor earlier that week for a pain in his back that had been bothering him for a while and the doctor wrote him a script. My father-in-law is a guy who doesn't take Tylenol, never mind a prescription from a doctor, so he wanted to know what the pills were. He put them in my hand and asked if they were ok to take with wine. When I looked down in my hand, there they were, Vicodin 7.5/750's, the same pill I took on that August morning in 2008 that started a seven-and-a-half-year struggle to find my way back to recovery. At that same moment Diana's grandfather asked me if I wanted a beer, something he does every time he sees me, with no malicious intent. He's a ninety-year-old, off the boat Italian man who doesn't know the extent of my story. It's normally something I just laugh off with the rest of the family, but that day, in that moment, I just thought to myself, *what the fuck* ? I looked up at my wife and sister-in-law who both had that same *what the fuck look on their face,* and just shook my head and laughed. I politely declined the offer for the beer like I always do and handed the bottle of Vicodin back to my father-in-law, telling him he probably shouldn't take them with wine. I shrugged it off and assured Diana and Jen that I was ok. We sat down for dinner and the day moved on. It was a hot, humid, Sunday afternoon in 2019, August 3rd to be exact and Diana's parents invited us over earlier that day. It was a regular Sunday dinner combined with a celebration of our second wedding anniversary. On July 29, 2017 Diana and I got married in front of our closest family and friends at a beautiful resort in Tulum, Mexico. Chris, Marissa, Sean, Anna, Little Greggy and his fiancé Lydia, were all in attendance, just as I imagined it the day I watched Chris and Marissa exchange their vows six years earlier. It was just one of the blessings bestowed upon me since that dark winter day in 2016 that I decided to change my life.

I got up from the table to get a bottle of water from the kitchen and something happened. I saw the bottle of pills on the counter, and I got that feeling I had gotten many times before. The euphoric recall of an opiate caused the tightening in my stomach and the rush of adrenaline that I was so familiar with but hadn't experienced in a long time. Three and a half years of recovery, three and a half years of good recovery and that feeling just came back like it never left. I looked at those pills and every ounce of me wanted to take a handful and put them in my pocket. I knew he would never take them so I knew he would never miss them. Just like that my brain went into automatic addict mode. Fuck doing the right thing, fuck being honest and fuck everything I built back up since I got clean and sober. The feeling was overwhelming and Diana saw it when I got back to the table. She asked what was wrong and I just told her I was fine. I needed to stop thinking about it, so I went into the living room to hang out with my two nephews. Nicholas was about to be seven and Dom was four, and my relationship with them had blossomed into one of the greatest blessings in my life. Anytime I didn't feel myself, an hour with those two will bring me right back to center. That night however, even Nicholas and Dom couldn't get my mind off what was in that kitchen. I told Diana I wasn't feeling well and needed to leave. We got in the car, drove home, and well after Diana went to sleep, I sat struggling with my thoughts, the rest of the night. I knew I should call someone, but I told myself it was too late. Why should I bother someone this late at night ? It was an excuse I didn't even believe myself. There's fifty different people I could go to at any given time. I knew more than one who would've been up to talk me through my struggle. I have taken many a call late at night and not once did I consider it a bothersome task. The truth was I was too proud to ask for help. It was a big reason I relapsed the first time around. I didn't want people to think I was weak. I didn't want to show my vulnerability. It's dangerous place to be and I knew that if I didn't let go of this way of thinking, history would surely repeat itself.

I finally fell asleep and when I got up for work the next morning, the feeling was still there. I told myself if it didn't subside by the end of the day, I would make the call I so desperately didn't want to make. I was assigned to Brooklyn North for the day to oversee a cleanup of a homeless encampment in Bushwick. In December of 2018, after twelve years and four months as a sanitation worker, I was promoted to Supervisor. It was a step that I was hesitant to take, and one that came with a lot more responsibility. After much thought and discussion with family and friends, I decided it was the best thing for my future and I gave it a shot. It turns out I was a natural at the job and I loved doing it. I spent the first six months working in upper Manhattan and had just transferred back to Brooklyn a few weeks earlier. The ride to work was a struggle, feelings of fear, guilt and shame about the thoughts I was having flooded my body. Once I arrived at work I was so busy getting my crews together and paperwork in order, that I didn't have time to sit in my own thoughts. Once we arrived on scene it was a waiting game. The process is a multi agency effort, and we had to wait for all to be on scene before the cleanup began. The thoughts and feelings returned, yet I still didn't make a call. About an hour after arriving on scene, all the respective agency representatives arrived. The cleanup began and my thoughts once again shifted to the task at hand. It was then that God stepped in and did for me what I was so reluctant to do for myself.

As the cleanup moved along I started talking to the representative from the volunteer homeless outreach program that was on scene. Our conversation ranged from our respective jobs to what happened in the Met game the day before. He worked nights in the food industry as a line cook, hoping one day have a restaurant of his own. He worked for the outreach program on his own time, as a volunteer, because he was once too homeless. He was once a homeless drug addict and alcoholic who found his way into recovery five years earlier and this was part of his way of giving back. As soon as he told me that, I opened up about my own struggles, and we spent the next hour talking about addiction, and the dark places it took us. We also talked about recovery and how much better our lives were today than they were when we were in active addiction. I told him about what happened the night before and the thoughts and feelings I was struggling with. He didn't judge me, nor did he dismiss my feelings. He listened, he understood, and he talked me through them, giving me an example of his own struggles with the very same feelings. I didn't know this man, but we shared a common bond and that's what recovery is all about. At its very core, it is one addict or alcoholic helping another, through the process of identification. I never saw him before that day and I never saw him again. I don't remember his name, but I will never forget how he helped me that day. When the cleanup was over I shook his hand and thanked him for our talk. I called my sponsor on the way home and told him everything, I shared my feelings at the next three meetings I attended that week. I had man after man come and talk to me after each meeting and walk me through their own experiences, assuring me that I would get through it with the help of God and the program. I just had to trust the process and be honest.

I look back on that whole scenario as the point in time when my whole attitude and outlook upon life changed. I found my faith and because of that faith I can accept life and all that comes along with it, good and bad, for what it is, no longer worrying about things I have no control over. I found an inner peace that allows me to be comfortable in my own skin. I'm confident in everything I do, knowing that all I'm responsible for is my best effort, the rest is out of my hands. When I tell my story, people will often ask if I have any regrets. There was a time when I was full of regret and that regret kept me sick and suffering inside. Today I don't regret my past because I wouldn't be the man I am today without it. I look back on it and I speak about it often, but I don't let it define me. Today I am five years clean and sober. I am a husband, a son, a cousin, a brother, an uncle and a friend. I wake up every day and try to live life the best way I can, helping as many as I can along the way. I never had those feelings after that night, but if they do come again I know I can get through them. Until then I will not stress. By the Grace of God, I will keep living life, clean and sober, a day at a time, forever grateful and forever blessed.

The End.

Lightning Source UK Ltd.
Milton Keynes UK
UKHW020645291021
393035UK00010B/584